Invisible Enemy

Environmental illness and one woman's search for a cure

Faye Hueston

Author contact: info@fayehueston.com
fayehueston.com

ISBN-13: 978-1530567584
ISBN-10: 1530567580

FIRST EDITION: 2016 v6.6
This book is a revised version of *Silent Enemy* and contains updated material.

9 8 7 6 5 4 3 2 1

Colophon
Body text composed in Adobe Minion Pro 11/15. Titles in The Mix Expert Caps (Adobe) 17/20 >50. Book design by Alan P. Scott, Raleigh, NC.

In memory of Rachel Carson,
Who sounded the warning,
And of Dr. Max Gerson,
Who provided the cure.

WARNING

The author is not a licensed physician and does not present her experiences with medical treatment as a guide for patients in need of care. Do not attempt self-diagnosis or initiate treatment based on the content of this book. The experiences related here are unique to the author and are not offered as a substitute for a licensed physician's in-person medical evaluation, diagnosis, and recommended treatment.

Rarely has anything been accomplished except by the genius of a single man, fighting against the crowd.

—Voltaire

The most formidable barrier to the advancement of Science is the conventional wisdom of the prevailing group.

—C. H. Waddington

ACKNOWLEDGMENTS

I would like to thank my book designer, Alan Scott, not only for his skill but also for his patience with the many changes he was asked to make. Thanks, too, must go to Ermie Macknee for her infinite patience in proofreading the book both before and after the changes. To Bruce March I owe a special debt of gratitude for his last minute editing and valuable recommendations.

Also by Faye Hueston
Fanchon's Daughter: A Memoir

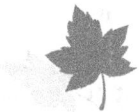

PROLOGUE

Many years ago while living in London, I became unaccountably ill. A mysterious process seemed to be at work within my body, undermining the vigorous health I had enjoyed for most of my life. This slow, imperceptible slide into infirmity alarmed me, for I was ill-prepared for sickness.

Raised as a Christian Scientist by my adoptive mother, I grew up in a Hollywood home that was affluent, pious, and teetotal. Believing illness to be a mere mental "belief," we saw no doctors, nor were there any medicines in our medicine cabinets. The only cure for a headache or a heart attack was prayer.

My adoptive father did not share our religion, although he respected it because of his deep mistrust of doctors—those "quacks" he never saw. While the connection between our faith and our genes may have been merely fortuitous, my parents, my adoptive brother, and I rejoiced in excellent health.

In 1963, my first serious illness brought me close to death. Saved at the eleventh hour by a doctor with antibiotics, and disillusioned with God and Mary Baker Eddy—both of whom I felt had let me down—I left the church. What I did not know was that my body still harbored the seeds of a future struggle—seeds that would not germinate for the next sixteen years.

I do not deny that spiritual healing is possible or that symptoms can, on occasion, be psychosomatically induced. My story, however, concerns a more prevalent situation in which prayer proves ineffectual and symptoms thought to be psychosomatic in origin, when correctly diagnosed, are found to have an environmental cause. Although my experience occurred some forty-odd years ago, it is even more relevant today.

As invasive chemicals multiply with great complexity in the world, they bring new and graver challenges for human health and survival. We are faced with an increasingly drug- and technology-oriented medical profession that is ill-equipped to deal with the subtle nature of environmental illness. One has only to consider the levels of pollution in our food, in our water, and in the very air we breathe, to realize the harm we are inflicting—not only on this planet, but on ourselves.

During the years when my health was declining and no one could tell me why, I thought I must be the only person on earth so strangely afflicted. Yet reason told me this couldn't be true; I was neither sinful enough nor saintly enough to have been singled out for some exotic torment. After the cause of my condition was found to be pesticide poisoning, I was led to the nutritional therapy that ultimately restored me to health.

Throughout this trial I was keeping a diary. Begun for the purpose of recording my dreams, some of which had proved to be precognitive, it became instead a record of the symptoms, setbacks, and occasional triumphs that accompanied my long and often discouraging search for a cure.

The following pages are a chronicle distilled from that journey.

CHAPTER ONE

I sensed something was wrong the moment I surfaced from the anesthetic. The feeling of an acid creeping under my scalp, and the pain that ran from one hip down the leg were new acquisitions. It had been my fifth operation within a year—this one to remove a silicone breast implant, following a mastectomy for cancer three months before.

Within weeks of the implant's insertion, my breast had begun to swell. Thinking I had an infection, my surgeon prescribed antibiotics. I had been given so many of these that year I was loath to take more, but having transferred my faith in God to faith in doctors, I lacked the courage to question their higher authority.

The first course of antibiotics failed, so my surgeon prescribed a second. When the swelling persisted, he proposed a third broad-spectrum course of the drugs. By then my breast felt like a balloon about to burst, so I demanded the implant be removed. A tissue sample was sent to the lab for culturing, but the report came back negative.

"Why, then, did my body reject the implant?" I asked the surgeon.

"I don't know," he replied. "It shouldn't have, because silicone is inert matter."

Little was known in the 1970s about the effect of silicone in the body, even when it was "safely enclosed" in a breast form. It didn't occur to me that the many drugs I had taken that year—tranquilizers, painkillers, anesthetics, and six courses of antibiotics—might have contributed to the implant's rejection. I only knew that between the time I entered the operating theater and the moment I regained consciousness in my room, something happened to my body that had nothing to do with the surgery on my breast.

Too drugged to think clearly, I assumed the symptoms would disappear, but they didn't; the sciatica lasted for almost a year. A friend who had been a nurse told me that patients under anesthesia were sometimes handled roughly while being transported from the operating theatre back to their rooms.

"It's not uncommon for minor injuries to occur," she said. "It's also not generally known that medical students are allowed to perform pelvic examinations on anesthetized women."

"*Pelvic exams!* Without our knowledge or consent?"

"That's right. Of course, you'd have a job trying to prove it in court, or to prove a minor injury such as yours. You can't touch the unions—or the doctors, for that matter. They all close ranks."

In the weeks that followed I became aware of a slight burning sensation in my scalp. Months later, my hairline began to recede. I consulted my National Health Service (NHS) doctor, a remote man I had met once before when my sixteen-year-old daughter came down with the flu.

"Well?" he said as I entered, raising his eyes from the papers on his desk. It was his only greeting. I ran through my repertoire of symptoms, to which he listened with all the interest of a mortician. When I described the peculiar crawling sensation under my scalp and the backward creep of my hairline, he rose, made a cursory examination of my scalp, saw no visible anomaly, and pronounced my symptoms psychosomatic.

"I know there's nothing you can see," I protested. "That's what's so puzzling."

"Have you thought of seeing a psychiatrist about this?" he asked.

"Why, no," I said, taken aback.

"I suggest that would be your best step," he advised, and returned to his desk. Since the visit seemed to be over, I said goodbye and left.

Dismissed as a hypochondriac by the National Health System, I turned to the private sector—a quest that took me through some of the costliest consulting rooms in London without bringing me any nearer a diagnosis or cure. At least the doctors I paid privately were too polite to say they thought I was mad. Instead, they fobbed me off with useless ointments, practiced smiles, and healthy bills.

A Sloane Street trichologist with impeccable manners examined my scalp and assured me the receding hair would grow back in the spring. Weeks later, a Mayfair specialist informed me my hair would never grow back. The only point on which the two experts agreed was that neither could offer a cure.

A third deity, a diminutive dermatologist in Harley Street with a large Arab clientele, had the honesty, or the chutzpah, to admit that no one really knows what causes hair to fall out. For this wisdom I received a bill larger than those presented by the other two. What a doddle this skin game is, I thought; all you need to charge the earth for your ignorance is an expensive education.

Weary of doctors who had no time for puzzling conditions—not even as an opportunity to hone their skills—I turned to the alternative field. The 1970s were a time of bold new approaches to health in holistic medicine. Disciplines such as the Silva Method and the Simonton's visualization technique stressed the integration of mind, body, and spirit in the healing process.

Exploring it all, I attended seminars given by self-styled gurus who jetted the world promising instant nirvana (for a price); joined a consciousness-raising group whose leader tried to bludgeon us into enlightenment; and met one or two souls who suggested that I look for the light within.

A guided meditation in a transpersonal psychology workshop had us climbing a mountain, at the top of which we would meet a wise old man who would tell us something we needed to know. The mountain appeared quite readily behind closed eyelids, rising from a meadow of yellow jonquils, its peak bathed in the violet hues of a setting sun.

Athrob with anticipation, I reached the summit but found no wise old man there ready to counsel me. I waited for him to appear, until the leader's soft voice instructed us to return our consciousness to the room. When we had all completed our inner journeys, we were invited to share the messages we'd received. To my chagrin, I was the only one to whom no wise old man had appeared. I was mortified, ashamed, my unworthiness confirmed.

A year later, in a different workshop, the same meditation was given and again I found myself on that mountaintop alone, waiting, and close to tears. This time, though, a wise old woman eventually appeared, but if she told me something I needed to know, I forgot what it was on the way down.

I tried Transcendental Meditation℠ but fared no better. Thoughts flitted and strayed, were brought under control, then scampered away again. Unwanted tunes kept playing in my head like musical tinnitus. My chattering mind could not be stilled.

Inspired by a book I had read on self-healing through visualization, I tried to envision my white blood cells attacking the enemy invader. But my condition had no name, hence no image that I could visualize, so I abandoned the effort.

Turning to the more practical end of the alternative field, I tried homeopathy, reflexology, osteopathy, iridology, kinesiology, acupuncture, and herbal remedies—each one for a period long enough to determine its efficacy, at least for me. On the whole, the practitioners I met were men and women of transparent dedication, each believing that his or her patch of the holistic field was the answer to most if not all of the body's ills.

"Your third chakra is unbalanced," said one therapist.

"What does that mean?"

"It means your stomach, liver, and nervous systems are out of balance. You need to be more grounded. And your yin-yang energy needs balancing as well."

To be sure, there were a few charlatans along the way, but they were easy to spot—as easy as were their conventional colleagues. Yet, wide though my net had been cast, by 1979 I was no better; indeed, I was getting worse. The fault, however, lay not with the therapies, for if they did not help, neither did they harm. Rather, the problem was that these disciplines evolved at a time when mankind was cooperating with nature, instead of trying to subdue her—a time when the world was a simpler and purer place than it has since become. Sadly, they were no match for the invisible enemy that was insinuating itself into every cell of my being.

As my health continued to decline, I felt that I had been drawn into some dark wood where there was no path, no guide, and where no one had gone before. In *The Masks of God*, Joseph Campbell paraphrases Dante's adventure as the psychological journey that occurs in the middle of life, symbolizing crucifixion, death, and the descent into hell, the passage through purgatory leading ultimately to paradise and the adventurer's return to service in the world. Since I was fast approaching the descent-into-hell phase, the prospect of paradise seemed to have been lost indeed.

In January 1980, I applied to the NHS to change my general practitioner. The new doctor, a youngish woman with short-cropped brown hair and a brisk, impersonal manner, listened patiently as I explained that my problems had begun three years earlier.

"… and still no one has been able to determine the cause of my symptoms," I concluded.

"Which are?"

I gave her a well-rehearsed rundown of the pincushion scalp, the headaches I woke up with in the middle of the night, and the sick-all-over-feeling I woke with each morning. From the expression on her face I might have been addressing a sphinx.

"Yes," she said, "I'm familiar with these symptoms. They're emotionally caused. Have you thought of seeing a psychiatrist?"

I blinked. This woman knew nothing about me. She hadn't even received my records from the former GP, whatever *they* contained. Yet within minutes of meeting me, she had concluded that my illness was psychological—as though incipient hair loss in a healthy middle-aged woman had merely an emotional cause. If that were so, by forty we would all be bald.

I returned home more discouraged than ever. It wasn't that no one understood what was wrong with me; it was that no one cared enough to *want* to understand. Of course it is easier for the busy doctor to consign a difficult patient to the psychiatrist, even though it was not that long ago that psychiatry itself was viewed with sniffy disdain. No matter; if the answer eludes pathology, the psychosomatic interpretation can always be trotted out (Freud has a lot to answer for). And if, on hearing the word "psychosomatic" for the *n*th time, the patient feels the teeniest urge to scream—well, that just proves the case, doesn't it?

No doubt there *are* those whose illness is self-generated, but I was not one of them. Raised in a religion that views illness as "a manifestation of erroneous thinking," I was more inclined to deny disease than invent it. Yet, even if we are the author of our woes, by what process does the mind create unwanted illness in the body? If disease is so easily acquired against our will, why is it so hard to get rid of when we consciously seek to be well? I had put this question to a number of practitioners, but answer came there none.

As for my symptoms having an emotional source, I had never been happier in my life. I had moved to London in 1970 after a divorce in Paris, I had two young daughters I adored, and I was in a relationship with someone who shared my love of literature and music. Moreover, I had no financial worries, thanks to my generous adoptive parents, which gave me the time to work on a book I was writing about my remarkable mother and my search for birth parents.

Physically, however, my problems were multiplying. Arthritis was interfering with the yoga I had practiced for seven years. When I rose from my desk my knees crunched like gravel, and when I woke in the morning, my neck, which I had injured when young, felt like a solid block of pain. At night, I would wake with a pounding headache or a teeth-chattering chill that sent me scurrying for a sweater, even in summer.

These symptoms, and the accompanying panic attacks, seemed like harbingers of menopause, but there were none of the more definitive signs. Moreover, my sickly flushes differed from the nighttime sweats of a menopausal friend. Beginning at the base of my spine, they rose in a sickening wave to my head, where they imploded like a silent madness in my brain.

What made these episodes so frightening was the sense of a loss of parameters, of there being no edge to hold onto. It was like losing my mind while remaining sane enough to feel every step of the disintegration process. As my benighted body relinquished one aspect of health after another, I felt betrayed, the way a great beauty must feel betrayed when her perfect features begin to wrinkle and sag.

The condition was also affecting my relationship with my teenage daughters, who were 14 and 16 at the time. Since there was no visible cause for my claims of illness, they viewed them as suspect and me as the most tiresome of mothers. And who could blame them? The search for health had taken over my life.

In the silent war being waged within my body, an attack could come at any moment. It could manifest as a tingling in my feet or a fibrillation of my heart or a sudden "chaos of the mind," the phrase Lord Byron used to describe his spells of manic depression. I had also become hypersensitive to noise. The slam of a door or the cry of a child in the street below was like an assault on my central nervous system.

One could hardly devise a more diabolic torment than one in which the victim is subject to forces no one can see, and has symptoms for which no cause can be found, while outwardly appearing to be perfectly well. Such a condition, if imposed on a criminal, would be considered cruel and inhuman punishment.

George Eliot, in *Middlemarch,* observes that "If we had a keen vision and feeling of all ordinary human life, it would be like hearing the grass grow and the squirrel's heart beat, and we should die of that roar which lies on the other side of silence." At times the inrush of sensory data resembled that silent roar—inaudible to others, yet overwhelming me with its noise. What had I done? Who had I wronged that I should be punished this way?

By May 1980, a year of acupuncture had failed to relieve either my headaches or hay fever. Homeopathy and herbal treatment also had failed. Yet I knew people who had been helped by these procedures. Why hadn't they helped me?

Advice came from every quarter, all of it well-meaning, most of it wrong. One doctor told me my problem was hormonal, another said it was too much acid, while a third diagnosed an infection. The rest insisted it was all in my mind. One healer told me "You're blocked," another said I was "too open," while a third said "Your aura is as full of holes as Swiss cheese." At the end of three years I had seen so many doctors, healers, and therapists, I wouldn't have known who to credit if I got better or who to blame if I grew worse.

As my symptoms increased, so did my frustration, for I knew they were not psychosomatic; they were *somatopsychic,* a case of the body influencing the brain. I knew this because my body kept telling me they were, and I had learned to listen to its wisdom.

Often during this period, a moment from childhood appeared in my mind's eye, as though it had been caught on a loop of film. I saw myself, aged eight or nine, running across the lawn of our Beverly Hills home thinking *How strong I am! I shall always be strong like this. Why should anyone be sick? If I'm ever sick, I shall simply will myself to be well!*

Knowing only health, I assumed it was my legacy for life. Nothing could harm me; I was invincible! Such arrogance of the fittest must have angered the gods, for one bent down just then and whispered, "Mark well this moment, child, and the health of which you are now so certain, for the memory may return one day to haunt you."

The mere blink of a moment—as evanescent as all the other moments long forgotten, yet it embedded itself in my mind like a fly trapped in amber, waiting to mock me now—now that I knew how impotent is the will in the face of illness.

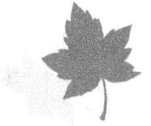

CHAPTER TWO

In December, the therapist to whom I submitted my arthritic joints for a monthly kneading advised me to walk for an hour each day. "Strong, purposeful strides," he ordered. "Sitting too long at your desk is part of the problem." So I strode through the nearby park, savoring the stillness and the new-fallen snow, but after three months my legs were no better. Something unwonted kept sapping my strength.

To be afflicted with the infirmities of age while still relatively young seemed an egregious affront. There were things I meant to do with my life—productive, outreaching things, such as writing and being of service to others in some way—not waste it in this endless preoccupation with my body. There *had* to be an explanation for what was happening to me, if only to prove wrong those all-knowing doctors who kept telling me my symptoms were psychosomatic. How did they know? How could they tell when they weren't living in my skin?

By April '81, I was dragging myself out of bed in the mornings, feeling ancient and feeble and depressed. Hobbling about on aching feet, I went to see a foot reflexologist I knew who lived in a third-floor walk-up off the Bayswater Road. Too weak to skip up the stairs as before, I pulled myself up by the handrail, step by slow, heavy step, the muscles in my legs as useless as spent rubber bands.

A year had passed since I'd last seen Joe and now, stretched out on his bed, with one aching foot resting in his lap, I said, "I hope *you* can tell me, Joe, why I'm falling apart."

Joe dug silently at my big toe with an iron thumb, while I dug my fingers into the bedspread to keep from howling. After a few moments he said, "Your adrenals are completely drained."

"What does that mean?"

"I'm not sure. Have you been under any stress lately?"

"I've scarcely been without it," I said. "But I don't believe in stress as a causative agent. Most people are under stress of one sort or another."

"Well, something is stressing your body," he said. "The trouble is in your lower spine."

"Then what can it be?" I persisted, aching for an answer, *any* answer. "I've never had back pain, and stress alone can't account for this wasting away of my strength."

Joe's thumb addressed other points on my toes.

"Are there any stressors in your personal life?" he asked.

"None," I replied. Indeed, my primary stress was being told that my symptoms were all in my head and that I needed to see a psychiatrist.

Along with the quest for health, I had been searching for something that could fill the spiritual void left by my departure from the church in 1963. After I moved to England I began to explore different forms of spirituality in the hope of gaining some insight into life's infinite perplexity. It was the sort of search one undertakes in one's twenties, not one's forties, but I had a lot of catching up to do. Yet now, when my need for inspiration was greatest, the number of sources who inspired seemed to be dwindling.

On the night of April 12, 1981, I had a dream with such transcendent imagery that it changed forever my sense of this waking world as the only world there is. I suspect that to each of us is granted, if only once in our lifetime, an intimation of something beyond the now that we know. However brief the vision, once it is glimpsed our sense of reality can never be the same.

The dream—although it was more than a dream—began in the waiting room of a doctor or healer. Here there occurs a hole in my memory, for on waking, the next thing I remembered was leaving the office by a different door and walking through a gray corridor that led to the street.

As I stepped onto the pavement I glanced down—and found that I could see right through it into its transparent depths. Tiny points of light were darting about in the velvety blackness beneath my feet. Surprised, I raised my eyes and saw that the world around me was suffused with a golden light unlike any I had ever seen. It did not merely illumine; it *permeated* creation with a pellucid, numinous glow.

I seemed to have left our three-dimensional world and stepped into one where every atom and particle could be seen through the solidity of structure. The surfaces of things had thinned, and I could see right through them into their very essence.

"Oh!" I heard myself gasp, "*This* is reality!" I had never seen it before, yet I recognized it instantly, as though from some far memory predating my existence. Engulfed in a kind of cosmic homesickness, I yearned to share the vision with someone—for, strangely, there were no people in this wondrous landscape.

I turned and rushed back to the waiting room, hoping for no rational reason to find my daughter Kate there, but the room was empty, and seemed even bleaker after that crystalline world outside. As I stood there, crestfallen, a silent voice seemed to say, "You don't understand; the vision can't be shared. You must experience it alone."

For a moment I felt bereft. But then, fearing the vision would vanish because I had turned away from it, I hurried outside—and there it was, a transparent world still glowing with incandescent beauty.

In May, as my condition worsened I went to see a Scottish healer I knew. I had met Bruce MacManaway shortly after moving to England, at one of

the weekend seminars he gave occasionally in London. Tall and imposing, a former major in the British Army, Bruce taught subjects such as
telepathy, extrasensory perception, and dowsing, better known as water
divining—all of which were new to me at the time.

I had never been interested in the so-called paranormal—nor, for
that matter, in ghost stories, science fiction, or romance novels. Fact,
not fiction, engaged me. Yet I relished a new experience, so when a
friend invited me to the seminar, I readily agreed.

Bruce told us he had discovered his healing gift while serving in
France during the Second World War. Finding himself in the field,
with a severely wounded comrade and no medical assistance, he had
felt impelled to place his hand on the soldier's open wound. To his surprise, the young man's pain quickly abated, as did the effects of shock.

"This happened again," said Bruce, "too often to have been mere
coincidence. As a result of these experiences, I decided after the war to
devote my life to healing."

By the time I met him in the '70s, Bruce was spending most of his
time teaching and training healers at his home in Scotland. Seated before him that day in London, hoping he could help me as he had helped
others, I tried to suppress the skeptical part of my mind.

"Well, now, Faye," he said, removing a pendulum from his pocket
and letting it swing between us, "what seems to be the problem?"

The pendulum was Bruce's only diagnostic tool. He asked *yes* or *no*
questions mentally, and the direction of the pendulum's swing indicated the answer. As I watched the bob move to and fro, I wondered how
to frame my reply. There were so many problems I didn't know where
to begin.

"Well, for a start I can't sleep. I keep waking at two in the morning
with a headache, my joints are stiffening, and my hair seems to be falling out. I feel exhausted much of the time, which isn't like me at all, and
I think I'm going mad. Shall I go on?"

The pendulum began to swing in a clockwise direction. "Have you
had your flat checked for noxious energies?" he asked.

"No. Why?"

"I think you may have a black stream running through your property." The swing grew stronger. "If I were you, I would find a good dowser to check this out. I would do it for you, but I'm returning to Scotland tomorrow."

I had learned from Bruce's seminars that "black streams" and "noxious energy fields" were two of the terms dowsers use to describe earth's fractured energy lines. These lines, which are not ley lines, form part of earth's planetary design, rising like invisible walls of energy from deep within its depths—how high we do not know. Although benign in their natural pattern, if the lines cross a polluted stream or become split, their effect on sensitive people can be malefic.

I promised Bruce I would find a dowser to vet the flat, although it was hard to believe that something as nebulous as an invisible energy could be causing my very tangible symptoms. Bruce then turned his attention to my spine, resting his hands on my lower back for several minutes before consigning me to one of his trainee healers, who went on to do most of the healing work.

Seating me on the massage table, she placed her hands gently on my back just above the shoulder blades. A lovely warmth began to suffuse my being. I thought of the many healers to whom I had submitted my hapless body, each time hoping that this person or that therapy would bring the longed-for cure. Yet I think I knew that whatever was wrong with me, it would not be cured by a simple laying-on of hands.

As soon as I reached home, I rang a friend I knew to be collaborating with a writer on an anthology of the paranormal. The term covers a broad range of phenomena, of which dowsing is mistakenly thought to be one. Dowsers, however, view the ability to obtain information through a faculty beyond the five senses as one that we all possess. This "sixth sense" has fallen into disuse as the distractions of civilization clamor ever more loudly for our attention—estranging us from our own inner knowing.

"Ruth," I said, "would you know of a dowser who specializes in earth energies? I think I may have a black stream going through my flat."

"I do, actually," she replied. "There's a retired wing commander in Maidenhead who is considered an expert on the subject. His name is Clive Beadon, and he's a former president of the British Dowsing Society. You can probably get his phone number through the Maidenhead exchange."

I reached Clive Beadon the next day.

"I'm afraid I can't help you at the moment," said the oddly high-pitched voice on the telephone. "I'm leaving for Arizona tomorrow, to find water in the desert for an American company. I'll be gone for about ten days, but if you can send me a map of your property, I'll have a look at the problem when I get back. I'll ring you when I can come to London and check things out on site."

The idea of consulting a map of my flat to determine if an invisible energy line went through it would have seemed the height of lunacy if Bruce hadn't also included in his seminars the phenomenon of map dowsing. Improbable though it may seem, any skilled dowser wishing to locate a source of water or an underground pipe or any other hidden object on a property, however distant, can find it as easily on a map of the area, using a pendulum, as on the site itself. Why this should be so, not even dowsers can explain. That it works is proven when water is found within a foot of where it was located on the map, and the dowser collects his fee.

The fact that a mere representation of a property can yield information about that property beggars belief. Its implications for our Euclidean concepts of image and space are mind-boggling. A map dowser works with the paradox that things must not only be seen to be believed, they must also be believed to be seen.

In 1933 Alfred Korzybski wrote, in *Science and Sanity,* "The map is not the territory." Apparently, Korzybski was wrong. In the strange world of dowsing, the map *is* the territory.

CHAPTER THREE

Clive Beadon, DFC, was the very model of a 1940s wing commander. Tall, mid-sixties, with ginger brows bristling above blue eyes, he
was wearing a brown blazer, its RAF buttons gleaming like bright little
badges of authority. Not until after his death did I learn from his obitu-
ary of the wartime exploit for which he was awarded the Distinguished
Flying Cross:

> In 1944, during a low-altitude attack on Japanese supply
> trains on the Bangkok-Chiang Mai Railway, the tail section
> of his plane was set ablaze and its gunner killed by Japanese
> antiaircraft fire, yet he managed to guide his crippled bomber
> more than 1,000 miles back to base.

He was standing as if at attention when I opened the door, a briefcase in one hand, a wooden box tucked under his other arm. Faintly
awed, I invited him in. He placed his briefcase and box on the hall table
and we exchanged the customary civilities.

"Now then," he said, addressing me in those clipped pukka vowels I'd
heard on the telephone, "I'd like to show you what I found on your map."

He snapped open his briefcase and removed the blueprint of my
flat that I had sent him. Spreading it out on the table, he explained,
"I've marked only the major lines here, but there are many more." I
peered at the map—now so crisscrossed with lines it looked as though
chopsticks had been scattered throughout the rooms. "As you can see,"
said Beadon, "it's a very disturbed situation you have here. In fact, I
haven't seen so many lines going through a property before."

"What do they mean?" I asked.

"We'll discuss that in a moment," he said. "But first, I would like to do a quick dowse of the flat, if I may."

He turned to his briefcase and withdrew a whalebone divining rod—also called the Y-rod because of its shape. Next, he opened the wooden box to reveal a warren of compartments containing curious objects: small vials filled with mysterious liquids, polished gemstones of various colors and shapes, several pendulums, and a plastic disk made of Perspex, about three inches in diameter and divided into eight equal sections, each of a different color.

Selecting the disk, Beadon palmed it in one hand before grasping both ends of the rod and setting it in the horizontal "search" position. He paused for a moment lifting his head as though harking to something. Shifting the disk slightly in his hand, he placed his ring finger on one of the segments and took several steps forward, saying, "Now there should be a red line about … here." At the word "here," the rod rose to a perpendicular position. Beadon brought the ends of the rod together to break the hold, set it again in the search position, and moved into the corridor, murmuring, as though to himself, "And another line … about here." Again the rod rose, as if on cue.

Beguiled by the thought of invisible lines that answered to color, I followed him as he walked through the rooms, the rod rising and falling as he went. I longed to ask what the disk was for, but didn't, for fear of putting him off his stride. Besides, Beadon was slightly intimidating.

He ended the dowse in the sitting room, placed the rod and disk on the coffee table, and, turning to me, said, "Now then, as I observed, your situation here is a very disturbed one. Frankly, I'm not surprised you've been having so many health problems."

"Before you tell me what I'm longing to know," I said, "do let me get you a drink."

"Thank you, my dear—a gin and tonic would be lovely."

I went to the kitchen, while Beadon fetched my map from the hall and spread it out on the coffee table. When I returned, he set the drink aside, picked up his rod, and using it as a pointer explained:

"Now—for a start, you have a polluted stream running diagonally under your bed, about seventy feet down. You also have five energy lines crossing through the bed here, about where your chest would be when you sleep. Some of these lines also traverse the stream, which can't have been doing you much good either. The negative influence of these energies is increased when they cross a polluted stream."

"Then you think *they* could be causing my symptoms?" I said, trying not to look as skeptical as I felt.

"I'm almost sure of it," he said, picking up his drink and sinking into the sofa.

"It's hard to believe my headaches and stiffening joints could be caused by something as nebulous as sleeping over a polluted stream," I said.

"Not 'caused,' " Beadon corrected me, "exacerbated. These energies can increase geopathic radiation, which is what this is called. They can also disrupt the metabolism of plants as well as people. Unfortunately," he added, "the average person is not aware of this—nor, for that matter, is the average doctor. Of course," he sniffed, "the medical profession keeps saying it needs more than anecdotal evidence, yet when proof is offered, it is dismissed out of hand."

"Well, you must admit that words like 'black streams' and 'invisible energies that respond to color' do invite a certain skepticism."

"Of course they do. Nonetheless, everything in nature identifies itself by color, even when the color is invisible. Now this," he said, reaching for the disk, "is divided into eight colors—or six, if you discount the black and white sections. It's called the Mager Rosette, after the Frenchman, Henri Mager, who created it, but I call it the color wheel. When searching for water, if you hold the wheel in your hand thusly, with your index finger touching the blue or white segment, your rod will respond only to potable water. Brackish or polluted water responds to gray or black, which may be where the term 'black stream' comes from."

"I had no idea dowsing could be so complicated," I said. "I've tried a few experiments with the pendulum, but I still don't understand how it works."

"Neither do I," said Beadon, cheerfully, "it just does. And frankly, I'm not much interested in theory. Success in dowsing is based on intent and visualization. If one's intent is focused, the unconscious kicks in and one's dowsing becomes more accurate.

"For example," he continued, "to find a vein of water you must think deep into the earth and visualize a running stream. It can be quite a narrow one, but it should be flowing through granite rock. Oddly enough, still water, such as a lake or a pond, doesn't emit these radiations. The reason it helps to use color when trying to distinguish a stream from an energy line is because the latter is picked up on red or yellow, whereas the stream is picked up on blue.

"Now, your problem," he added, "appears to be that you react unconsciously to these energies, which is why you have been troubled by the stream and the lines that cross through your bed. So you'll need to learn how to control your sensitivity."

He paused, studied me for a moment, then said, "I say ... given your sensitivity to these energies, I might use you as a guinea pig for the control I'm working on."

"What sort of control ..." I asked, my interest quickening.

"To shield people from the harmful effects of geopathic stress. I've been trying to find a better way of neutralizing these energies than the methods that have been applied hitherto, which is why I developed the spiral."

"The spiral?"

"The name I've given the control I'm working on—'The Spiral of Tranquility.' However," he added, glancing at his watch, "I'm afraid I haven't time to go into that now; I have to be in Maida Vale at four."

The stab of regret I felt at his leaving surprised me. It had been a long time since my mind had been so captured by a subject. As we walked toward the hall I said, "Well, I do hope you can do something about these energies, whatever they are."

"I'll do my best," said Beadon, with the sort of smile that did not countenance failure. "Now, I'll try to have a control ready for you in a week or so. In the meantime, if you would like to try to find the stream yourself, I can leave my rod and color wheel for you to play with. Oh, don't worry," he added, "I always carry an extra set with me."

He closed the box, snapped his briefcase shut, and swept both off the table.

"Well, goodbye, my dear," he said. "I'll ring you when I'm next in London."

I waited at the door while he pressed the bell for the lift. Six floors down its ancient gears ground into action. Too impatient to wait for its poky ascent Beadon took the stairs, and with a wave of his hand disappeared behind the lift shaft.

I closed the door, reflecting on the strange new world that had just opened up to me. How did it happen that water, my friend since childhood, had become an enemy when polluted, even when I didn't know it was there? And if dowsers had to search for a polluted stream, why was I unable to escape its noxious radiations?

Curious to see if I could find the stream Beadon said ran under my bed, I picked up his rod and color wheel and went to my room. Placing my ring finger on the black segment of the disk, as I had seen him do, I walked slowly toward the foot of the bed trying to visualize a narrow stream running through granite rock deep in the earth. As I neared the corner the rod began to rise, as though an unseen hand was pushing it up from below. I traversed the foot of the bed and the rod relaxed, resuming the horizontal position. When I proceeded up the other side, however, the rod rose again when I neared the headboard. This seemed to confirm Beadon's description of the stream's diagonal path.

But was I really picking up the stream or had I let his description influence my mind? Could the mind alone have created the powerful force I had felt pushing up against the rod?

Reflecting on the interaction of image, energy, and thought, it occurred to me that if we can find a polluted stream simply by visualizing it while thinking deep into the earth, what might we not discover by thinking high into the heavens—by tuning in to the infinite, so to speak, or to cosmic consciousness or God or universal mind or whatever one wants to call that mysterious power that sometimes works wonders in our lives?

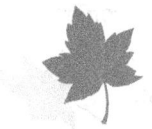

CHAPTER FOUR

In the weeks following Clive Beadon's visit, I grew rapidly worse. At night the stream's radiations invaded my body, draining my strength and stiffening my joints. When I walked in the park the earth rejected me with its mold and the trees with their pollen. How could I live in a world where even nature had turned against me? Only the flowers greeted me when I passed, yet even some of these—the most fragrant—sickened me with their scent.

My body felt like a patchwork of quivering flesh, flinching at every shift in the environment and reacting to every toxin in the air. Even my heart had abandoned its normal rhythm, skipping a beat one moment and speeding up the next. I nearly fainted in Harrods one day when it suddenly paused, then began to thump so violently against my chest I thought it was going to stop. Days later, an electrocardiogram showed my heart to be perfectly sound.

Beadon delivered his Spiral of Tranquility in mid-June.

"Sorry I couldn't get this to you sooner," he said, removing a small box from his briefcase and handing it to me. "My wife has been ill—she has a bad heart—and the jobs have been piling up. I'm afraid I can't stay long," he added, declining a drink.

I opened the box to find an acrylic block two inches square with a copper spiral embedded in the center, surrounded by a number of floating gemstone chips.

Entranced with its oddity, I asked, "What are the gemstones for?"

"Well, dowsers have known for ages that copper can divert some of these negative energies from a property, but I found that copper alone doesn't do the whole job. This troubled me, so I looked for a method that would take care of the rest."

"What made you think of gemstones?"

"I don't know why it occurred to me to experiment with crystals, but I found that certain stones, if placed at the point of entry on a map of the property, will block these lines from the property itself without sending the problem on to someone else. One must take great care when attempting to change the environment. By adding the correct stones to the copper, the control seemed to achieve better staying power."

"I see," I said, not seeing at all how crystals and copper could thwart a determined energy line.

"Now I'm going to leave this control with you," said Beadon. "As long as you keep it in the open on a wooden surface—not glass, glass will fracture the lines—it should deflect both the energy lines and the influence of the stream. I'll ring you in a few days, and you can tell me if things have quieted down."

The flat did feel calmer for a day or two, but then the telltale symptoms began to creep back. When Beadon rang for his report, I had to convey the disappointing news.

"How tiresome," he said. "I shall have to rethink the situation in your flat."

His next spiral produced the same effect: palpable relief for forty-eight hours, followed by a gradual return of the energy lines. Once, when Clive was testing a control on my map in Maidenhead I felt an uncomfortable pressure in my lungs. Wondering if it could be caused by one of the stones, I rang him at home.

"Absolutely not," he replied. "If you were going to be bothered by a crystal you would have felt it before now." But then he noticed he'd left a malachite stone lying on a corner of my map on his desk. When he removed it, the pressure in my lungs eased. This surprised Clive as much as it did me.

"You're a very queer fish, aren't you?" he observed, his voice tinged with annoyance.

Another time, he inadvertently left a small mirror lying across one of the energy lines on my map, which fractured the line in my flat, prompting another emergency call to Maidenhead. When he removed the mirror, the same relief ensued.

The third time this happened, Clive remarked, "You're absurdly sensitive to crystals, aren't you."

"I'm absurdly sensitive to *everything*," I replied, grimly.

There was a slight pause at the other end. Then, "I say, there's something I would like to try. Do you have your pendulum handy? Good. Now, don't hang up. Go stand in one of those energy lines by your bed, pick up the phone there and let me know what the pendulum's doing."

I did as he instructed, positioning myself by the telephone on my bedside table.

"I'm standing over the stream now, Clive," I reported, "or maybe it's an energy line, I'm not sure which…."

"Doesn't matter. Pendulum going around? Fine. Now I'm going to do something to your map here, and I want you to tell me if the pendulum changes its swing."

I watched the bob as it slowed and adopted a clockwise course, wondering what Beadon could be doing to my map in his study. The swing then began to decelerate.

"It's slowing down, Clive," I reported. "Wait … now it's still. What have you done?"

"Never mind. Just tell me if it starts up again."

Which it did. This game—for that's what it seemed to me at the time—continued for twenty minutes or so, the pendulum spinning in one direction, slowing down, then reversing its spin or adopting a diagonal path—all, apparently, in response to something Beadon was doing on a map of my flat miles away. I could not have been influencing the pendulum's movements, since I had no idea what he was up to or why.

Eventually, he said, "I think I may have found the stones that will take care of your problem. I'll make a mock-up control and bring it round when I'm next in London."

This was the first of what would become six years of long-distance dowsing experiments in an effort to shield me from the energies in my flat. Each time a test spiral failed—and each one did after a few days—Clive, undaunted, returned to the dowsing board.

Once, when he was in London, he said, only half-jokingly, "I can't understand why you're such a problem; none of my other clients give me such a hard time."

"That's because I'm not a client anymore," I retorted, "I'm a guinea pig, and your guinea piggery is giving *me* a hard time."

He shot me a rueful look. "Well, if I can block you, I can block anyone."

Much as Clive relished a challenge, he was finding the problems in my flat more vexatious than he had bargained for. As the months wore on and one disappointment followed another, the strain began to tell on us both. For Clive, it meant more work on my flat when he had important jobs to do and dowsing seminars to prepare. For me, it meant an ever-deepening discouragement.

One day in September, after another test spiral had failed, he said, "You know, given the pernicious nature of these energies, you might want to think about moving."

"Moving!" I exclaimed, "Never!" The mere thought was so stress-inducing I refused to consider it. *"I will not run away from this problem!"* I wrote in my diary that night, with the sense of writing my epitaph. Meanwhile, I was growing feebler by the day and no one could tell me why.

In October, hard calluses began to form on the soles of my feet, sores appeared on the roof of my mouth, and rashes broke out on different parts of my body. There were nights when I woke with an inchoate fear and the feeling that my sanity was slipping away. What in God's name was happening to me? I wondered. If only I knew. If only *someone* knew.

In December I considered abandoning the book on adoption and writing about this experience instead, but a book about an illness with no name, no known cause, and no cure at the end? It was hard enough to live—it would be impossible to read.

When I had to go to New York for a week, my symptoms abated to some extent, which lent credence to Clive's conviction that the cause of my problems lay in my flat. The evening before my return I attended a dinner party, where I indulged in my three worst addictions: chocolate, coffee, and cheese. I had always prided myself on being able to eat anything, but that evening, as my hands turned scarlet, I suspected this was no longer the case.

Proof came the next morning, when I woke feeling as though a steel rod had been rammed through my skull. By the time I reached the airport I was in agony. No alcoholic hangover could rival the pain that throbbed in my head during every second of that interminable flight back to London.

By March of '83, the calluses on the soles of my feet had spread to the heels. When my right foot developed a lingering pain, I went to see the doctor I had managed to avoid since our first meeting. She was away, so I saw her locum instead—a breezy young man who was seeing patients as though sizing eggs on a conveyor belt. He examined my foot and dismissed the pain as unimportant.

"But what if it gets worse over the long Easter weekend?" I asked.

"Well, it will just be Murphy's Law then, won't it?" he said, cheerfully.

"Murphy's Law?"

" 'If things can get worse at the worst possible time, they will.' "

"That's not very reassuring," I said.

"That's life," he shrugged.

That's the caring NHS.

Days later, an X-ray of my foot failed to reveal any cause for the pain. Gazing at its skeletal image I was reminded of the times my mother took me to Bullocks Wilshire to buy my clothes for school. The children's shoe department had a wonderful toy: an X-ray machine! If you slid your feet through an opening at the bottom and looked down through a window, you could see the bones in your toes as clear as could be. When I think of all the minutes I spent wiggling my toes in those hazardous rays, it's a wonder that cancer didn't find me before I reached my forties. How many roentgens were absorbed by young bones before those machines were finally removed in the1960s? How many adult cancers might be traced to those lingering childhood exposures?

In April, there were nights when the energy lines were so strong I couldn't stay in the flat and had to doss down with a sleeping bag in the home of an indulgent friend—only to find that *her* environment was almost as disturbed as my own. Why, then, didn't *she* feel these energies, too?

How strange I must have seemed to my friends then; how strange I seem to myself now. Yet my distress was not imaginary. It was as real as if someone had plugged me into an electrical socket and set the current on high.

By mid-April the soles of my feet were so sensitive I could scarcely bear the pressure of shoes. Going barefoot at home, I kept stubbing my toes, and managed to break two. When, oh *when*, would I ever walk again without pain?

Eventually, I gave in to Clive's repeated suggestions that I move. After all, I reasoned, "to move" did not necessarily mean to run away; it could also mean to go forward. Having thus rationalized my compliance, in May 1983 I began to search for another flat.

I found one in an old building that was being renovated on Onslow Square. Before committing to it, however, I told the estate agent I would like to have a friend see it first. Accordingly, Clive met us there on the appointed day and did a walk-through dowse of the rooms. Trotting along behind him with my own rod and color wheel, I caught sight of the agent's face, which seemed to be saying, "Crikey! I've got a couple of right Charlies here!"

"Well", said Clive, folding his rod, "the bedroom is clear. I can find nothing here that should disturb you."

With this assurance, I took the flat and booked the move for the first week in June, wondering how I was going to manage all the packing in my debilitated state. With the help of a friend I moved a mattress into the empty flat and slept on the floor until the furniture arrived. It felt a bit spooky at night, being alone in the building with no telephone—there were no cell phones then—and no way to call for help if an emergency arose.

With the move only a month away, the demands on my diminishing strength increased. When wall-to-wall carpeting was installed in the flat, I became so ill that night that I thought I was going to die. If I did, I reflected, I would have died without knowing what had taken my life.

Two days later, I tripped over some tools in the hallway left by a carpenter and broke another toe.

The move to Onslow Gardens proved to be a triumph of necessity over infirmity. The calluses on my feet had developed fissures that were starting to bleed, and by the end of the month a dark crust had formed over the weeping soles. It was like having the stigmata on one's feet while lacking the strong religious faith that would have given them meaning.

One night, I was invited to the private screening of a documentary about a young man afflicted with *ichthyosis vulgaris*. This is a hideous disease that causes the surface of the skin to become rough and scaly, like the scales on a fish. The man's back and arms were black from the dirt that had collected in the crevices, which bore an alarming resemblance to the fissures that were forming on my feet.

The film followed the attempt of a hypnotherapist to cure the condition through hypnotic suggestion. Remarkably, he had succeeded in restoring part of the young man's epidermis to its normal state. But then a doctor informed him that ichthyosis is a congenital disease, and therefore incurable. From that moment on, the therapist could no longer influence the condition.

The fact that ichthyosis is hereditary should have forestalled the morbid fears that were forming in my mind, since I knew enough about the health history of my birth parents, by then, to dispel such imaginings. At the time, however, I could not help wondering if the crusts accreting on the soles of my feet, like barnacles on a ship, could be the first stage of this rare and disfiguring disease.

CHAPTER FIVE

In September I learned of a Dr. Choy at the Wellington Hospital who was studying the effect of electricity on sensitive people. I reached him on the phone and he suggested that I see his colleague, Dr. Monro. "She's very interested in problems like yours," he said.

The receptionist at Dr. Monro's office handed me the customary new patient questionnaire. This one, however, was unlike any I had ever seen. In addition to the usual queries about past illnesses and operations, it asked about my home environment: What sort of cleaning products did I use? What type of cooking and heating fuel—gas or electricity? Were carpets, curtains, and furniture coverings made of natural or synthetic fibers? Simply by having to think about these things for the first time, I became aware of them in a way that I hadn't been before.

Dr. Monro turned out to be an attractive young woman with fair hair swept into a twist and a voice as soft as a young girl's. Beneath this gentle exterior, however, lay a spine of tempered steel—and Jean Monro needed one, for pitted against her was the British medical establishment, as hostile to unorthodox medicine in England as the American Medical Association (AMA) is in this country.

She studied my questionnaire, lifting her eyes at times to inquire about a particular symptom, as though it was significant rather than imaginary.

"I hope you don't think my symptoms too weird," I said.

"Not at all," she replied. "We're quite open-minded about things here."

Dr. Monro thought my problems could be caused by allergy and suggested we do some testing to determine my "frequencies"—whatever those were. "For the moment," she said, "the testing procedure is being done at my home in Kings Langley, while we complete negotiations for space in another hospital in London."

She gave me an appointment, with directions to her home in Hertfordshire, and I left her office with a new, if cautious, feeling of hope. I liked Jean Monro. She had none of the self-importance of some of her male colleagues. Even if her treatment failed, it would be an interesting experience.

I arrived at Dr. Monro's home in early October, only to be brought up short by a notice on the front door:

IF YOU ARE WEARING PERFUME, COLOGNE, OR HAIRSPRAY, OR IF YOU SMELL OF TOBACCO SMOKE, PLEASE DO NOT ENTER. RING FOR THE NURSE.

No one had warned me. I had dabbed a touch of cologne on my wrist that morning—it was a habit I had all but abandoned. The thought that I had come all that way, only to find I could not be tested, was disheartening. I rang the bell. A nurse came to the door. I explained my predicament and she went to fetch Dr. Monro.

"I'm so sorry," said Dr. Monro. "You should have been given these instructions in advance. We have some very sick people here who are highly sensitive to chemicals. If you don't mind washing off your perfume with soap in the upstairs bathroom, you can stay. You'll find a cotton shirt hanging there on a hook, which you can put on afterwards, because some of the scent may still be clinging to your blouse."

I went upstairs and scrubbed the offending cologne from my skin, keeping a watchful eye on the spider poised at the edge of the sink. After donning the shirt, I returned downstairs, but before I could enter the testing room, I had to pass a "sniff" test by the nurse.

There was only one patient there—a young woman in her thirties, whose feet were so deformed with arthritis, they made me wonder what mine would be like if the calluses grew much worse? The cracks in my heels had become so painful the only shoes I could tolerate were sandals, yet even in these I walked with the tread of a leper.

The nurse returned with some long narrow boxes labeled "wheat," "corn," "molds," "house dust mite," "monosodium glutamate," and so forth.

"These are antigens," she explained. "An antigen is a substance capable of stimulating an immune response. Each box contains ten vials filled with homeopathic doses of a single antigen suspended in a saline solution. Homeopathy is a system of treating diseases with minute doses of a natural substance that, in healthy people, would produce symptoms similar to the disease. Of course, all the foods used in these antigens are organically grown."

"How does the treatment work?" I asked, intrigued.

"The vials are numbered 1 to 10. The higher the number, the weaker the antigen. The testing procedure, called 'skin titration,' involves injecting a dose of the antigen into the skin of the upper arm in serial dilutions." The nurse took a vial from the box and inserted a syringe. "These intradermal injections produce a raised wheal," she explained, injecting the dose into my arm, "and we always start with Wheat #2, because wheat is one of the most common allergens."

A wheal quickly appeared on my arm. Taking a small ruler from her breast pocket, she measured its size, then set the timer on the table for ten minutes. "When the timer rings," she said, "I'll measure the wheal again. If it has grown, you're deemed sensitive to the substance and a weaker dilution, #3, will be injected. We continue this procedure until the neutralizing dose—or 'end point'—is reached. That's the amount that does not provoke a symptom or increase the size of the wheal."

"And the neutralizing dose stops the reaction?"

"It neutralizes reactions to foods, pollens, chemicals, and any other substances the body regards as hostile. This allows it to build up its immune system so that future encounters with these substances can be tolerated. Of course as the patient improves, the end point changes, so retesting is periodically required."

While she was speaking, Dr. Monro entered the room and continued the explanation.

"Patients are rarely sensitive to just one group of antigens. In some patients, reactions will occur chiefly to chemicals, while in others it will be to foods or inhaled particles. However," she cautioned, "the desensitizing drops act slowly and only if allergenic foods are eaten in moderation. The drops do not protect against binging, nor do they cure addiction. They control symptoms."

I was to record the antigen number and any symptoms that occurred during the ten-minute interval. None appeared, but when the timer rang the wheal had grown, so the nurse injected Wheat #3 into my arm. Within minutes my legs grew stiff, my hands turned crimson, and a wave of heat surged through my body. This continued until we reached my end point of #7.

Noting my scarlet fingers, the nurse took hold of my hands and turned them over to inspect the palms. "You certainly are allergic to wheat, aren't you?" she said.

"I'm certainly addicted to it," I confessed, "but how can I be allergic to something I eat every day?"

"That's called 'masked allergy,'" she explained. "It masks as an addiction. Withdrawal from the food produces the same sort of craving smokers have when they're deprived of a cigarette. The body struggles to adapt to the allergen by producing symptoms that have no apparent relation to the substance itself, and because we are all different, each patient may react differently to the same substance."

The concept of allergy as addiction was new to me. If true, I thought, it might explain why doctors, who diagnose from symptoms, can be confused by conditions that don't conform to a known pathological pattern. After all, they can't diagnose what they don't know exists.

"At the end of the session," the nurse continued, "your end-point dose will be placed in a dropper bottle to be taken sublingually four times a day. For patients with multiple allergies, ten antigens can be combined in a single dose for self-injection."

It soon became evident that testing was a time-consuming business, especially if one reacted strongly to a substance and required successive injections. More patients had arrived by then, and I fell into conversation with the pretty young woman sitting next to me. Her name was Amanda and I discovered that she was one of Dr. Monro's earliest and sickest patients. Her story was so unusual it had been written up in the papers, which is where many of Dr. Monro's patients first learned about her practice.

"When Jean found me two years ago," she said (all Dr. Monro's patients called her Jean), "I was a 'universal reactor'—you know, sensitive to everything in the environment—what the papers like to call 'allergic to the twentieth century.' My hair had fallen out, and I was so discouraged that twice I tried to end my life.

"Jean put me up in an old trailer here in her backyard, with just a bed and cotton curtains at the windows. I lived in it for a year while she treated me. The trailer had to be old," Amanda explained, "so that all its toxic odors, like formaldehyde, had outgassed. The only clothing I could tolerate against my skin was a cotton shift, and the few things I could eat had to be brought to me from the kitchen, because I couldn't touch metal cooking utensils."

It was hard to believe Amanda could ever have been so ill, for her hair was now long and lustrous and she was able to lead a normal, if cautious, life. Most of the people in the room that day were leading lives of quiet desperation. It was like finding I belonged to a club I had no wish to join, but of which I had been an unwitting member for years. Invisibly maimed, we were a fellowship of freaks. Our symptoms may have differed, but the process that had brought us there was the same: the long, discouraging search for a cure that kept leading to skeptical doctors and the dead end of psychogenic dismissal. If some of us were allergic to the twentieth century, I thought, maybe there was something wrong with the century.

I had noticed the nurse referred occasionally to a book that lay on the corner table. I asked her about it.

"It's called *Allergy: Your Hidden Enemy*, by Dr. Theron Randolph," she said. "Dr. Randolph is the father of clinical ecology. Every doctor and every allergy patient should read this book." I glanced through it and decided to pick up a copy on my way home.

Settling down with Randolph's book that evening, I had read no further than the dedication when I knew that its author was the kind of doctor I had been hoping to find.

> This book is dedicated to all patients who have ever been called neurotic, hypochondriac, hysterical, or starved for attention, while actually suffering from environmentally induced illness.

At last; someone who understood, someone who had risked the scorn of his colleagues in order to help those whom they had abandoned. Hungrily, I read about hidden addiction, the chemicals in our food, the pollution in our air, the poisons in our water, and the price we are paying for our reckless disregard of nature. I learned that the questionnaire I had filled in for Dr. Monro was the one Randolph had devised for his patients in Chicago. I learned that many hyperallergic people grow sicker gradually over a period of years through small, incremental exposures to environmental toxins, and that a preexisting condition can be made suddenly worse by a massive exposure to an allergy-causing substance.

What, I wondered, could my preexisting condition have been? A fragile immune system? An unknown genetic inheritance? When I met my birth mother in '77, I discovered that she had suffered from the same hay fever she had passed on to me.

I recalled a friend saying, "Isn't it odd, Faye, that you lead such a healthy life—I mean, you don't drink, smoke, or do drugs, and you eat all the right things, yet you have such peculiar physical problems?"

It was true. A fish-eating herbivore, I lived on vegetables, fruits, and nuts, ate only whole-meal bread, drank only bottled spring water and decaffeinated coffee (later, a coffee substitute), and took all the requisite vitamins, minerals, and herbs, yet my maladies multiplied, while friends who drank, smoked, and ate the most appalling junk food seemed to thrive. Except that two later died in their fifties of colon cancer.

What I didn't know then was that plastic bottles leached their plasticizers into the spring water; that the caffeine-removing process left traces of methyl chloride in the coffee; that my coffee substitute was composed of grains to which I was allergic; and that the binding material of most over-the-counter vitamin pills is wheat or corn—grains again.

Worse, my healthy fruits and vegetables were not as healthy as I supposed, because they were sprayed with organophosphates, the most toxic of which, DDT, though banned in England and the US, was still being exported to third-world countries, who returned it to us on their heavily sprayed imported produce.

Allergy was a trickster. How could I be allergic to food when I never had heartburn, when I ate shellfish with impunity, and had a headache only if I drank two glasses of wine? I now understood why wheat made me sleepy, why fats gave me flushes, and why my "hypoallergenic" soap made me sneeze.

Admittedly, environmental illness is not a winning complaint. A Camille sneezing with hay fever instead of coughing with consumption would have been a pretty rum heroine, and as for Armand, he'd have had a job sustaining his passion as she wheezed with asthma through blocked bronchial tubes.

How different it was when I had cancer. Then, friends rallied round, all sympathy and solicitude, their concern informed by a mixture of fear and identification: *This could happen to me!* Cancer is serious. With cancer you can die, and death is respected. But no one dies of an allergy—do they?

I could only bless the fate that had led me to a doctor who saw in my symptoms—not a psychological disorder, but the lineaments of environmental illness and a collapsing immune system.

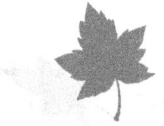

CHAPTER SIX

"Before I sign this," said Dr. Thorne, pen poised over the document I had presented, "I would like to know something about the procedure you want me to authorize."

It was my first meeting with the new NHS doctor to whom I'd been assigned after moving to Onslow Gardens. I rarely used the National Health, but I needed his signature on certain forms to authorize Jean's treatment.

A tall careful man in his thirties, Dr. Thorne was only marginally less remote than his predecessors. But then, I had come to expect wariness from doctors when they learned I was using alternative methods in addition to theirs.

I explained the skin titration procedure, but could tell from the way his jaw began to work that he was not in a receptive mood. When I described the sense of an acid crawling under my scalp and the sudden rush of heat to my head, he pursed his lips.

"I see," he said. "Are you sure you're not creating your illness unconsciously in order to gain sympathy at home?"

How does one answer such a question? *Why, of course I am, doctor. It works a treat every time!*

"No," I said evenly, "I'm a single parent, and there's no one at home from whom sympathy could be gained." Indeed, when my daughters were home from school, they were too absorbed in their own affairs to give much thought to me—let alone sympathy.

Dr. Thorne reflected for a moment, then signed the paper with evident distaste. I thanked him for his courtesy and left, reproaching myself for doing such a bad job explaining Jean's treatment.

His remark about creating my own illness, however, reminded me of the dermatologist I'd heard on the radio, who bemoaned "patients who faked their allergies." He accused them of subverting what would have been "effective treatment"—his, presumably—by "taking drugs, creams, and things they know they shouldn't." "Dermatological pathomimicry," he called it—confirming my suspicion that for some doctors, blinding us with bunkum beats solving the problem. It was our old friend blame-the-victim again, dressed up in highfalutin' medico-speak to explain away failed treatment.

On impulse, I stopped at a bookstore and bought a copy of Randolph's book to give to Dr. Thorne. I left it at his office the next day, with a note saying I hoped he would find the subject of interest. Well, he did say he wanted to know something about the procedure.

"Have you removed the control from your flat?" Clive demanded on the phone. "I've just checked your property on the map here and it appears to be off."

"I had to put it in a drawer, Clive. Something was bothering me last night and I wondered if it could be the Spiral, so I put it away to see if it made a difference."

"And did it?"

"Not really."

"Then put it back."

My flat had few secrets from Clive. He had only to swing a pendulum over my map in Maidenhead to know whether my environment in London had changed. Intriguing though this was, such long-distance surveillance was disconcerting. I didn't fancy him peering into my bedroom whenever he liked with his bloody pendulum.

Occasionally, when I returned home, I would find a message waiting for me on my answering machine:

"Just to let you know I've been watching this new control overnight and it looks promising, over and out." Or, "I think I've found the small problem that's been bothering you. I'll be having a shot at it this morning. Ring you later, over and out."

Old wing commanders never died. At least this one hadn't given up on me yet. My body, however, appeared to be doing just that.

In November, Jean's practice moved to the Nightingale Hospital in Lisson Grove. By then, the antigen testing had produced some surprising results.

Three days after the test for avocado, the wheals on my arm still looked like angry spider bites, and with the first injection of lettuce—a daily staple—I felt spaced out. This spaciness persisted until I reached the end point of #10. It was my strongest reaction to date, although the weakest attenuation of the antigen. The nurse refused to let me drive home until she had given me the "turn-off remedy"—a combination of potassium, baking soda, and vitamin C in eight ounces of water that neutralizes most allergic reactions.

On the fifteenth, I began testing "the nasties," the most frequently found chemicals in the environment: phenol, terpene, formalin, chlorine, ethanol, glycerol, Dacron®, polyester, and nylon.

"We're going to start you on mixed papers this morning," she said, preparing the syringe.

"Why papers?" I asked, rolling up my shirt sleeve.

"Because of the chemicals in ink, newsprint, and all kinds of paper," she explained, injecting Papers #3 into my arm.

"Oh, dear, all the things I work with every day. I suppose they're in typewriter ribbon as well?"

"Of course. Almost everyone who is allergic to foods, pollens, or molds also reacts to these chemicals, although not all in the same way."

As if to confirm her words, when I took the morning paper from my handbag, the patient next to me said,

"Would you mind putting that away? It's the chemicals in the newsprint, you see. I'm affected by the smell."

I quickly returned the paper to my bag, wondering why I hadn't thought to question the dark smudges it left on my fingers each morning. The patient's reaction, however, reminded me of a passage I had read in James Erlichman's *Gluttons for Punishment:*

> Humans can be ten times more sensitive than animals to toxic chemicals, and in addition, some humans are ten times more sensitive than others.

One woman in the room was so sensitive her neutralizing dose was off the chart—somewhere in the 200s, an attenuation so weak it amounted to the merest memory of a substance. The only way she could be tested was to place successive drops of an antigen on the back of her hand until she reached the dose that turned off her symptoms.

Watching her do this, I exclaimed, "Why, that's similar to dowsing!"

"Dowsing?" she said. "What's that?"

"What you're doing—reacting to something so subtle it can't be measured or seen, like the trace of a toxin."

"Oh," she said, not very interested. My timer went off then, and the nurse came to measure the wheal on my arm. By the time she'd injected me with papers #4, the conversation had moved on.

Another woman with strong chemical sensitivities could not be tested by injection, either, because she was allergic to the nickel in the needle. Instead, she held each antigen vial in her hand until she reached one that did not produce a reaction. In other words, the smallest trace of a chemical substance suspended in a saline solution, when merely held against her skin, produced the same effect as if it had been injected.

"My worst reactions were to chlorine," she told me. "It caused terrible headaches and exhaustion and the feeling of being utterly drained."

I thought back to my childhood, whole days of which had been spent in a chlorinated swimming pool, gulping down great mouthfuls of the stuff. When I watched the pool man dump buckets of chlorine into the water, I never imagined that it could be harmful—even though it made my eyes sting and stay bloodshot for hours after a swim.

The more I observed the reactions of my fellow patients, the more I was struck by the similarity between allergic sensitivity and the dowsing response, though with one important difference: The allergy sufferer reacts unconsciously to a substance he may not even be aware of, whereas the dowser needs to tune in *consciously* to whatever he is seeking to obtain a response. In each case, however, the reaction is to something so subtle it can't be measured scientifically or explained.

I was moaning about this sensitivity to a friend one day, when she remarked, "Do you know what you remind me of? *The Princess and the Pea.*"

We had a good laugh over this, for in truth my predicament was almost as absurd as that of Andersen's hyper-delicate princess. How was it possible that I, in my bed on the sixth floor, could feel the radiation from a polluted stream seventy-odd feet under the ground? How could the real princess have been kept awake all night by a pea hidden under seven mattresses, while the common pretend-princess slept soundly in her bed? What a gullible goose the queen must have been to think the heroine's hyperesthesia proved her royal blood, when in fact she was just a girl with a broken-down immune system.

I met many such princesses at the clinic—women who were affected by things far less tangible than a pea. In the testing room one day, we were startled when a patient cried, "I smell smoke!" This prompted a worried rush to the window. When no sign of smoke was seen, we returned to our chairs and the nurse did a sniff test of the room. To my chagrin, the culprit turned out to be my lapsang suchong tea, which I had just decanted from a thermos—its smoky aroma having reached the patient seated at the farthest end of the room.

Such an extreme acuity only increases the sufferer's sense of isolation. After all, a *visible* disability at least elicits compassion. No one tells the MS sufferer she has willed herself into a wheelchair to gain sympathy, or the polio victim that his paralysis has been self-induced. Yet the chemically sensitive person must contend not only with her illness, but with the skepticism of friends and the suspicion of doctors that she is not quite right in the head. Small wonder if we are driven to despair—not by our affliction alone, but by the blank incomprehension of our fellow men.

The discovery of how inimical to health are the smallest amounts of chemicals in our bodies brought a radical change to my way of life. Standing in the supermarket one day, I realized that on all those tempting shelves there was almost nothing I could safely eat—nothing that did not have colorings, additives, fillers, or preservatives. The tins were lined with phenol; the drinks were in plastic bottles (another phenol hazard); and every product that was boxed, packaged, or frozen contained added sugar or salt. We cared more for the shelf life of our food than we did for the lifespan of our bodies. Even the labels could not be trusted, for manufacturers were not compelled to list certain ingredients that only a few people are allergic to. Nothing was safe. For the chemically sensitive, the supermarket was a minefield.

I recalled another radio dietitian who declared, "There is *no* evidence whatsoever that chemicals, colorings, or preservatives in our food do us harm."

When doomsday arrives and we are all keeling over from toxic overload, no doubt the penultimate voice to be heard in the land will be that of a government spokesperson assuring us "There is no immediate danger," followed by a doctor, psychiatrist, or dietitian telling us "It is all in our minds."

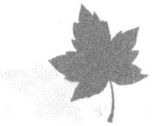

CHAPTER SEVEN

While testing for more nasties at the clinic in November, the first injection of nylon sent a fiery pain shooting through my arm. My fingers throbbed and my heart thumped so violently, the nurse had to give me the turn-off remedy again.

Something odd happened during this session that I am still at a loss to explain. There were five of us in the small room that day: four women and a man. I was sitting next to the corner table, on which was stacked the boxes of chemical antigens we were to test that day. The Dacron box was lying open on top, its ten vials exposed.

Seated cater-corner to the table on my right, were a man and a woman. Another woman sat opposite me, reading a book, while the two women on my left were engaged in conversation with the nurse. She was the only one on duty that morning, though there should have been two, so the testing procedure was taking even longer than usual.

Impatient with the delay, it occurred to me that if I could dowse for my end point, it would save time and I could avoid those pesky pricks in the arm. I glanced around the room. The man and woman on my right were engrossed in their books, as was the woman directly opposite. The two women on my left were still chatting with the nurse.

I reached furtively into my handbag and withdrew my pendulum. Suspending it from the fingers of my left hand, I rested my right palm on the exposed vials of Dacron while asking mentally, *What is my end point number for Dacron?* I was absorbed in counting the bob's rotations when I heard a voice say, "Put that pendulum away at once!"

Startled, I looked up to see the nurse glaring at me while administering the turn-off injection to one of the women. "You must *never* use a pendulum where sensitive patients are being tested," she said, angrily. "I *wondered* why these patients went suddenly into reaction."

To my astonishment both women appeared to be in some distress, for which my innocent dowsing was being blamed.

"But they *couldn't* have been affected by what I was doing," I said. "I wasn't even thinking about them; I was only trying to find my end point for Dacron. Besides, this pendulum is just a piece of plastic. It has no power of its own."

"You may think that it doesn't," retorted the nurse, "but it does. We've had this happen before when someone has used a pendulum near sensitive patients."

"But *I'm* sensitive, too," I protested, "and it hasn't hurt me. I don't see how it could possibly harm anyone else."

"Well, it does," said the woman nearest me, who appeared to be the most affected. "That's why our symptoms flared so suddenly."

"Nonsense," I said, "you weren't even aware of what I was doing."

"That doesn't matter," snapped the nurse, rubbing the woman's arm with an alcohol swab at the site.

There ensued a heated discussion among the four women—the man tactfully abstaining—as to whether the pendulum could create a disturbance simply by virtue of its swing, a view I hotly denied.

"It can only respond to the thought and *intent* of the dowser," I insisted, "and as my intent was innocent, and my thought focused only on myself, I don't see how it could have affected you or anyone else—for good *or* for ill."

"Oh, but it's a well-known fact that the pendulum creates a magnetic field," chimed in the lady opposite me.

"Rubbish," I said, refusing even to dignify that canard by challenging her source. "It can't 'create' anything. It simply registers whatever the subconscious mind is picking up at a given moment. If others imagine themselves to be affected, it must be due to suggestion."

"Not so," protested the woman on my left, pointing out that her back had been turned to me at the time, so suggestion didn't enter into it.

"I didn't see what you were doing, either," added the nurse, "until the change in these patients alerted me to the fact that something had happened."

To all this I listened in bewildered disbelief. It wasn't possible my innocent dowsing could have affected anyone, yet it appeared to have done so. Appalled at the thought of harming anyone, I put the pendulum away and apologized—although for what, I didn't know.

Some time later, Dr. Choy entered the room and came up to my chair.

"I'm afraid I must ask you, please", he said, in his polite Chinese manner, "not to use the pendulum when you're in the hospital. I was with a patient on the floor directly above when she took a sudden turn for the worse and asked me if someone in the hospital was using a pendulum. I said 'no' because I didn't know you had done so until I returned to this floor and the nurse told me what happened."

I was speechless. How could my use of a pendulum have affected someone on another floor whom I didn't even know? It wasn't the distance I doubted, for distance means nothing in dowsing, but intent *does*, and my intent had been innocent. Mortified, and more bewildered than ever, I apologized again and buried my head in a book for the rest of the session.

I rang Clive as soon as I reached home.

"... So there it is, Clive. What do you make of it?"

"Absolute rubbish!" he snorted. "In all my years of using the pendulum and reading about it, I have never heard of such a thing happening. It is nonsense to think you could have affected anyone other than yourself."

"I know. That's what I told them. And yet it happened."

That evening, while recording the incident in my diary, a strong chemical odor appeared in the room, the way the scent of perfume sometimes hovered briefly over my desk when I wrote about my mother. When this happened, I liked to think it was her spirit visiting me, for we used to joke about the heavy floral perfume she favored, which I disliked.

That night, however, the odor was of paint stripper or nail varnish. Was I going mad, or had my olfactory nerves become so sensitive that life on this planet would soon be impossible?

Two days later, while discussing the incident with Dr. Monro, she told me about an experience she'd had a year earlier that led her to ban the use of a pendulum in her clinic.

"A healer was brought in—with the patient's consent, of course— to measure the level of something in her body, using a pendulum. Suddenly, the patient went into a coma and it took me three weeks to nurse her back to health. So you see," she added, "I do know that such things can happen."

In the days that followed I kept turning the incident over in my mind, trying to find a explanation. A possible, if not wholly rational one occurred to me.

Each of us in the room that day shared a co-sensitivity to chemicals, which the testing procedure would have intensified. Conceivably, we might have interacted on some unconscious level. My hand had been resting on the doses of Dacron suspended in a saline solution, and we know that water is a conductor of energy.

Could my weak permeable immune system have absorbed the homeopathic dilutions and transmitted their combined energy in some way to the women sitting nearest me? Earlier, I had experienced a fiery reaction to nylon; perhaps the addition of Dacron created a toxin so volatile it reached the highly sensitive women on my left.

But if that was the case, what kind of energy were we dealing with? Why wasn't *I* affected as well? Why weren't the other patients in the room affected? And how are we to explain the reaction of the woman on the floor above?

The more I tried to find a logical explanation, the more incomprehensible the incident became.

And so it remains to this day.

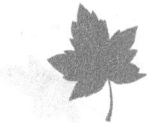

CHAPTER EIGHT

Three months into the allergy treatment, the pain in my foot was gone and the crusts on the soles of my feet were starting to heal. I hadn't had a sneezing spasm for weeks, and my eyes had stopped watering when house dust mite was added to the antigens. So subtly had these changes occurred I scarcely noticed them, pain's remission being less startling than its onset. I was now injecting the vaccines, as I had too many to be taken sublingually. Still worrying, however, was the state of my hair, which would go limp for long periods, then mysteriously regain its curl.

While contemplating my strong reaction to the nylon antigen, I recalled the way my body rejected the silicone breast implant in 1974. In 1980, with a view to reconstruction, I had asked the surgeon to insert a tiny piece of silicone in my midriff. If it still caused a reaction I would abandon the thought of reconstruction. In the event, it didn't, but something told me not to risk the operation.

Now, however, I wanted the piece removed—assuming it could be found—for small though it was, it was still a foreign substance in my body. My surgeon had since died, and the tiny scar had disappeared, so I consulted a Harley Street practitioner as to the feasibility of the procedure.

Mr. Naylor, as I shall call him—all surgeons in England are called "Mr."—was tall, slim, impeccably groomed and insufferably condescending. As elegant as the silk foulard in his breast pocket, he was all courtesy and unctuous charm—until he heard the word "allergy."

"Of course, I don't believe in allergies," he said.

"Why would my body have rejected the implant then if it wasn't allergic to the silicone?" I asked. It seemed a reasonable question.

"You do realize, dear lady," he said, as though addressing a dim chemistry student, "that silicone is an inert substance; therefore, you cannot possibly be allergic to it."

"Unfortunately, Mr. Naylor, I have learned that one can be allergic to almost anything."

He studied me coolly for a moment, his chin resting on long, elegant fingers. Then, "Have you considered seeing a psychiatrist about this?"

I thought I had become inured to this question, but I could feel the rage rising in my gorge.

"No," I said, biting my tongue.

"Why not? Are you afraid to see one?"

"No, I don't need to see one."

"How do you know you don't need to?"

"Are you implying that if I don't see a psychiatrist it's because I'm afraid to, and if I do, I'm admitting my problem is psychosomatic?"

"How do you know it's not psychosomatic?" he countered.

"How do you know that it is?" I shot back. "Have you seen this condition before?"

"Never."

"Then how do you know it's not allergy?"

He sighed and waved a limp hand—as though dismissing a tiresome witness from the stand. There being no useful purpose in prolonging the discussion, I was about to leave, when Mr. Naylor made what I can only describe as an improper suggestion.

"Of course I *could* operate on you, take a bit of silicone from somewhere and pretend that I found it in your body."

"And why would you do that?" I asked, trying to contain my contempt.

"Well, it would have the same effect, wouldn't it?"

I did not trust myself to reply. It was all I could do to muster a civil goodbye before fleeing his office. *And these are the men we encourage to play God!* I thought. Clearly, the clinic had been testing me for the wrong things. I should have been tested for doctor tolerance, ego tolerance, scientific-authority tolerance—and not on an empty stomach!

Driving home, I thought of a poem by another allergy sufferer. Yip Harburg was the Hollywood lyricist who wrote the lyrics for *The Wizard of Oz:*

> I'm really not hypochondriacal,
> Though the fear of a seizure cardiacal
>   Makes me jumpy and tense and maniacal
> With each inhalation of breath.
>   I'm really not hypochondriacal.
> I'm merely allergic to death.

The Christmas season brought a surge of social activity, making a shambles of my dietary resolve and turning the diary that was to record my dreams into a record of my recidivism. Binging on carbohydrates, I understood why the last indulgence granted the prisoner on death row is not sex, but food. If only gluttony had made me ill or given me spots or put fat on my frame, the goad of vanity might have restrained me, but I could lay waste a box of chocolates and have nothing worse to show for it than a guilty conscience and a sense of self-disgust. *That* was the sickening part of it.

Retesting my antigens at the clinic in January, I was sitting next to a weepy Amanda.

"What's the matter, Amanda?" I asked.

"I'm being tested for cow's milk," she snuffled, "and it always makes me feel depressed."

"You know, Amanda," said a patient, "I suffered from indigestion for thirty-four years, and the first day they tested me for cow's milk I found I was highly allergic. So I cut out all dairy products for two days and my indigestion disappeared. I haven't touched dairy since."

"But I don't eat dairy products," said Amanda.

A retired headmistress offered her experience.

"I had postprandial depression every morning for years and I didn't know why. When they tested me for honey, I became so overwhelmed with sadness I began to weep. I couldn't believe this healthy food I had been eating each morning for breakfast could be the cause of my depression. Had one of my girls at school behaved as I was behaving, I would have told her to snap out of it and pull herself together."

Amanda sniffed and made a little show of pulling herself together.

Throughout this conversation we heard muffled screams coming intermittently from an adjacent room. Now, suddenly, the door opened and a young woman emerged, whom I recognized as the engaging patient I had sat next to the week before. On seeing me, she colored.

"I hope I wasn't making too much noise in there," she said. "When I'm being tested for wheat I become so crazy they need two nurses to hold me down, so they have to test me in a separate room."

"Good heavens!" I exclaimed. "Do you react this way each time you eat bread?"

"Oh no, that's what's so odd. But I do have bad premenstrual tension, which wheat seems to exacerbate."

How interesting, I thought. Could it be that certain people, thought to be psychotic because of behavioral problems, were actually suffering from an unsuspected food intolerance?

I turned to Amanda:

"Why do *you* think some of us are allergic to so many things, Amanda, while others aren't affected at all?"

"Don't know," she sniffed. "Guess we're just more sensitive."

"Yes, but *why* are we more sensitive?" I persisted. "What has made us so?"

"Just born that way, I guess," she sighed.

But I was born normal; it was only in my forties I became a freak.

Of course, genetics had something to do with it, but that couldn't be the answer in every case.

Half a century ago Rachel Carson posed the same question in *Silent Spring*:

> What makes one person allergic to dusts or pollen, sensitive to a poison, or susceptible to an infection whereas another is not, is a medical mystery for which there is at present no explanation…. Some physicians estimate that a third or more of their patients show signs of some form of sensitivity, and that the number is growing. And unfortunately, sensitivity may suddenly develop in a person previously insensitive. In fact, some medical men believe that intermittent exposures to chemicals may produce just such sensitivity.

In January I saw Dr. Thorne again, since I needed his signature on some new forms for Jean. He signed them as distantly as before and returned them to me across his desk.

"Was there anything else you wished to see me about?" he asked.

"No, thank you," I replied. I did want him to know, however, that Jean's treatment was helping me, so I added, "In fact, I'm feeling much better."

This happy news haven elicited no flicker of interest or pleasure, I was about to leave, when I remembered the book I had left for him in October.

"Oh, by the way, Dr. Thorne, did you receive the book I dropped off for you after our first appointment?"

"I did."

I waited for him to say something. "Well … have you had time to look at it?"

"No."

"Oh." I murmured something about knowing how busy he was, but the tone of that "No" pricked my curiosity. "Do you think you will look at it, eventually?"

"I may dip into it—I may not."

"I don't understand. Why wouldn't you?"

"Because I prefer to study the subject in a more structured way, within the framework of my own discipline."

"I see. It's just that … I understand allergy isn't included in the syllabus at medical school—at least not in any depth—so I thought you might be interested in knowing something about the clinical ecology approach."

He fixed me with eyes as gray as a Gauleiter's. "I'm not interested in some new experimental therapy."

"But it's not new. It has been practiced for fifty years. Anyway, isn't every advance in medicine experimental at first?"

"Yes, well, that doesn't concern me. I take the view that I'm here to help you. You are not here to teach me."

I winced. That was *me* put in my place. But why had he interpreted my gesture as an affront to his authority? Didn't all good doctors learn from their patients? Jean did. Randolph did. What did it matter *where* knowledge comes from, as long as we keep learning?

Perhaps my lack of education wasn't such a handicap after all, if it saved me from having a single discipline into which things needed to fit. Unprejudiced by knowledge, I was free to make unorthodox connections. For some doctors, however, saving face seemed more important than opening the mind.

I could understand the hostility doctors feel toward methods that fly in the face of everything they were taught in medical school, for they have careers to protect and an expensive education to defend. To admit that some of what they learned could be out of date or even wrong requires a degree of humility not always compatible with their profession.

I thought back to the Sunday morning, weeks before, when the energies piercing through me were so unbearable that death seemed the only possible relief. After a long inner struggle, I picked up the phone and called Jean. Only desperation could have made me disturb her at home on a Sunday—yet instead of resenting my call, as she had every right to do, she responded immediately.

"Can you get here on your own or shall I send a car for you?"

"I think I can make it," I said.

Twice, on the drive to Kings Langley, I almost passed out and had to pull into a lay-by where I prayed for the strength to go on. When I finally reached her home, Jean was at the door. She led me into her kitchen, gave me the turn-off remedy, and took my vital signs, while I sat at her table feeling miserable and guilty for being there. After a while, when my symptoms began to ease, Jean left me to go to the next room. I heard her call Dr. Choy.

"Hello, Ray," she said through the open door, "I have Faye here, and…." I was too ill to hear what she was saying, but the one thing I do remember, and which has stayed with me all these years, is the curiosity in her voice, as though she were an anthropologist who had just received another peculiar specimen.

"Yes," I heard her say, "isn't it *interesting?*"

Returning to the kitchen, Jean said, "I can't let you drive home in your condition. I think you should spend the night here. You can sleep in the van. It's environmentally safe, and if we cover the windows with aluminum foil, you should be protected from the energies that are affecting you."

Jean fetched some bedclothes from the house, while her son brought a mattress to place on the floor of the van. Then he drove into town to get some heavy-duty foil to tape over the windows. The foil was useless, as I knew it would be, since not even a Faraday cage can block energies that pass through steel.

That night I spent in Jean's van remains the longest night of my life. Each second was more agonizing than the last. I thought of Amanda and the year she had lived in Jean's trailer. Had she, too, known the same physical torment? Did she, too, fear she was losing her mind? But no, this lucid torment was worse than madness. Oh, make me mad, I prayed, so that I may no longer feel! Had I not been near the one person who cared—the only one on earth who understood and was trying to help—I'm not sure how the night would have ended.

Recovering my wits in Thorne's office, I said, "We seem to be at cross purposes, Dr. Thorne. In view of the way you feel about the treatment I'm receiving, perhaps you would like me to find another doctor."

"Go right ahead," he said, with withering alacrity.

I left his office feeling more disconsolate than ever. How could a doctor—a *scientist*—be so incurious? Had *I* chosen to practice medicine, it would have been for the joy of discovery; of extending the boundaries of knowledge and proving there are *no* incurable diseases, only those for which the cure had yet to be found. I would have searched for that cure the way Jean was searching—not to gain wealth or honors or fame, but for the sake of helping those whom mainstream medicine had abandoned.

I drove to the nearest pharmacy and asked for a list of the NHS doctors in my area. The pharmacist, at least, was cordial and provided me with their names. Before I could apply to a new GP, however, I received a letter from the Kensington & Chelsea & Westminster Family Practitioner Committee, informing me that Dr. Thorne had told them he no longer wished to be my NHS doctor and had instructed them to remove my name from his list of patients.

So there it was, official and demeaning.

That night, as chemical goblins closed in again, I made a solemn pact with the Almighty: *Look, God, you can close as many minds as you like, only please—please close down my sensitivity, too.*

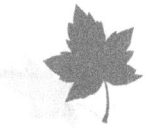

CHAPTER NINE

In June 1984 Jean learned about a new blood test in America that could identify the presence of any chemical in the body and measure the exact amount, utilizing gas chromatography and mass spectrographic analysis. Developed by a biochemist formerly with NASA, the technique could detect pesticides at levels as low as 0.1 parts per billion.

"This is an important diagnostic advance in the field of clinical ecology," Jean told me. "I think we should have you tested for chlorinated pesticides."

"Why pesticides?"

"Because recent studies on patients with possible exposure to pesticides have indicated that levels can remain in the body for as long as twenty years after exposure."

"Twenty years!"

"Yes, one part per billion appears to be the level at which clinical symptoms appear. So the relationship between chemical exposure and clinical symptoms exists at an exceedingly low level. Can you recall any exposures you may have had in the past?"

"Not offhand, no ... although, now that I think of it, when I was on honeymoon in Acapulco, we were having lunch by the pool one day, when a man began spraying the lawn around the tables and a fine mist fell over our food. I remember thinking, *He must be mad!* But we went on eating, so I guess *we* were the crazy ones.

"Oh, and each summer, when bugs and spiders crawl into my sitting room from the balcony, I've been killing them with a large insecticide spray gun. I loathe bugs, so I'm sure I spray them longer than is absolutely necessary. And then—oh Jean, I'm ashamed to tell you this—I've closed all the windows and continued to work at my desk, breathing those awful fumes for hours. I can't believe now how stupid I've been!"

Jean shook her head at such folly, but gave me a forgiving smile. "Well, it's not only insecticides," she said. "It's also organophosphates, which are commonly found in the home. These can cause fatigue, mental confusion, and short-term memory loss, in addition to depression and mood swings."

"All of which I've had, save for the mood swings."

"They can also cause tingling or pricking sensations," she added, "as well as numbness of the limbs."

"But if this is known, why are these chemicals still being sold?"

"Why indeed," she said. "Anyway, we'll have you tested to see if this could be your problem."

A Vacutainer of my blood was sent accordingly to the lab in Louisiana. The results would not be known for several weeks, but Jean felt they could be significant in forming a more complete diagnosis.

I had been reading Philip Toynbee's *End of a Journey*, the journal he kept when he was dying of cancer and wrestling with his Roman Catholic faith. "I thank God for all those genial hours in which He has allowed me to forget Him," he writes. Recalling my own struggle with religion in '64, I closed the book feeling at peace with my apostasy. *Thank God I'm no longer religious*, I thought. *And thank God I'm not clever enough to be complicated.*

The chemical profiles arrived in July, and Jean asked me to come in to discuss mine. As I passed through the glass doors of the Wellington Hospitals, I was suddenly reminded of something a clairvoyant once told me.

What led me to consult a medium was the sudden need to find my birth father, whose name I had just discovered in August of '74. He would have been seventy by then, and hoping clairvoyance might lead me to him more quickly, I obtained a sitting with the foremost medium in England. At one point, she gazed at an invisible screen beyond my right shoulder and said, "Now I see you going in and out of hotels with glass doors. Not *staying* in them, mind, but going in and out, in and out of glass doors."

This made no sense to me then. Why would I be going in and out of hotels without staying in them? As I passed through the Wellington's glass doors that day, however, her words came back to me. Clairvoyants can only interpret the symbols they see, and to a clairvoyant's eye the hospital could have been mistaken for a modern hotel. "We're not always sure if what we are seeing is the present or the future," I recalled her saying.

I reached Jean's office, eager to learn the results of my test. Referring to the report, she began:

"The analysis shows the presence of DDT and dieldrin, as well as a high level of heptachlor epoxide—a very toxic pesticide. Also high are your levels of beta-BHC."

"What is that?"

"It's a compound of benzene hexachloride that affects a wide range of enzymes. You also have hexachlorobenzine, which is found in pesticides, fungicides, and herbicides."

"Oh, no!" I said, hiding my face in my hands. "That wretched spray gun!"

"Highest of all, though," said Jean, "are the levels of DDE and DDD, herbicides which are derivatives of DDT."

"But how can that be? DDT was banned in the US years ago."

"It's banned in the UK, too," she said, "but these derivatives are returned to us on the heavily sprayed produce from third-world countries, to which they are still being sold." (Note: Paul H. Mueller, the Swiss chemist who developed DDT, received a Nobel Prize; Rachel Carson, who warned us about its danger, did not.)

"Then I must have consumed a ton of these toxins since '73, when I became a vegetarian."

"Your pesticide levels aren't as high as those for some of my patients," said Jean. "One man has levels that are literally off the chart, but you seem to be more sensitive to smaller amounts."

"But where could I have acquired all these other chemicals? The only one I know I was exposed to for years is chlorine."

"You could have absorbed them in a number of ways," Jean explained. "It needn't always be a strong exposure. The benzenes, for example, are found in dry cleaning fluid, and formaldehyde is found in anything from chipboard or particle board, to leather goods, to wall insulation."

"But if they're so pervasive, they must be impossible to avoid."

"I'm afraid so," she said. "Commercial products usually contain a combination of several chemicals suspended in a petroleum distillate, as well as a dispensing agent. Exposure to only one is the exception rather than the rule."

So, then, the cause of my illness was known at last: I had pesticide poisoning. My symptoms were not psychosomatic; they were *somato-psychic,* as I knew them to be all along. The only question now was how to get these toxins out of my system. And could this even be done?

That spring, a conference on allergies was held in London, at which Dr. Theron Randolph and Dr. William Rae, a clinical ecologist, were two of the speakers. The third was Dr. John Lassiter, the biochemist who had developed the chlorinated pesticide test.

Of the three, I found Dr. Lassiter's address the most compelling. A cautionary tale, it described the chemicals being found in the farthest reaches of the Arctic Ocean.

"We have put down our probes in the most remote parts of the ocean," he said, "and have found that even there no part of the sea is any longer free of pollution."

At a dinner given by Jean after the conference, I was seated next to Dr. Randolph, who proved to be the soul of avuncular warmth. Invited to lunch by Dr. Lassiter the next day, I confided in him my concern about the antigens, which no longer seemed to be working. Although the calluses on my feet had healed, some of my former symptoms had returned.

"Do you think a two-week stay at Randolph's ECU in Chicago would help?" I asked. "At least it would give my body a rest from the things I can't seem to escape here in London."

"If I were you I would go to Dr. Rae in Texas," Lassiter advised. "His environmentally controlled unit in Dallas has been modeled on the one Randolph created for his patients in Chicago. Rae is younger and has newer ideas."

Adding to my misery that spring were endless renovations being carried out on the buildings to either side of mine. Trucks dumped their loads onto the pavement, airborne toxins flew in through the window, and particulates drifted down through the chimney, leaving a delicate film of dust on the furniture.

As my health declined, the square outside my window was burgeoning with life. How I envied nature's ability to renew itself each spring. If the crocus and daffodil could regenerate, why couldn't my hair follicles do the same? Why was my hay fever the only thing that burgeoned? I *loved* Mother Nature; I worshiped every tree, shrub, plant, and flower She created. So why did she muck up my sinuses each spring with her pollen?

"Why don't you move to the country?" suggested Clive.

"And be poisoned by a farmer spraying his crops? No, thank you. I've moved once and that didn't help. It's no use, Clive. Unless I can get these chemicals out of my system, this problem will follow me wherever I go.

In July arrhythmic heartbeats began. They became so alarming one night that Jean sent me to the hospital. Tempted though I was to take the sedative they offered, I declined. If my heart was going to pack up for good, I wanted to be conscious, not comatose, when it did. Death was too important an adventure to sleep through.

On the 28th I was bedridden with bone-aching fatigue, a hammering head, and a heart that kept threatening to stop altogether. Clive rang for a report on his latest control and we had our first row.

"I think the new control is making my heart act funny, Clive, and my chest is feeling tight. Do you think the gemstones could be interacting with other crystals here in the building—in someone's jewelry, perhaps?"

"Nonsense!" he said. "I've had three different controls here for days, and they haven't bothered me a bit, so whatever you're feeling, it must be in your mind."

To hear from Clive's lips the same words I'd been hearing from doctors made me grind my teeth. How like him to assume that if *he* couldn't feel what was bothering *me*, it didn't exist—unless, of course, it began to bother *him!*

"But you know you're not as sensitive to crystals as I am," I pointed out.

"As for your heart," he continued, "I won't even consider that possibility unless you agree to see my wife's heart specialist in Windsor."

"But I don't *have* a heart problem, Clive. My EKG weeks ago was normal. This tachycardia must be a reaction to something—either some toxin in the flat or one of the crystals."

At this, a small explosion erupted at the other end. Open-minded though he was about most things, Clive was allergic to any criticism of his gemstone control.

"Anyway," I said, "I'm not going to waste more money on another specialist who will just prescribe Inderal® and charge me a whopping great fee."

"Then you will have to leave your flat!" he said, his high-pitched voice rising higher as the line from Maidenhead heated up. "I can't help you if you won't take my advice," he added in a voice that was even stiffer than his neck. "I only deal with the environment."

With that he rang off, leaving me with a knot in my stomach that stayed there for the rest of the day.

One morning, a strong chemical odor appeared in the bathroom. It faded after a minute or so, but reappeared in the kitchen that afternoon. The next day, I was awakened by the sound of clanging pipes at the other end of the flat. Throwing on a robe, I went to investigate. A scaffold was being erected outside my kitchen window. I raised the window and asked a workman what the scaffold was for.

"We're painting the exterior trim," he explained.

Two days later, vapors from an asphalt-making machine in the street made their way into my flat. It was the hottest day of the year, and I couldn't open a window because of the fumes. Even the *air* was unfit for human consumption!

The following morning, I was jolted out of bed by the sound of a pneumatic drill starting up outside. Stumbling to the window, I saw some men tearing up the asphalt in the same place they'd torn it up six months earlier. Every demolition crew in SW7 seemed to have descended on Onslow Gardens. Short of ripping up the square, I thought, there wasn't much more they could do.

I was wrong. There was.

That afternoon, they began resurfacing the street—the part they had just ripped up. Fumes from a simmering cauldron made their way into my flat, bypassing the air purifier I had bought to absorb them. Which of all these poisons, I wondered, will be the one to do me in?

The chemicals in the street? The gas-fired paint stripper a neighbor was using on her front door? Or her sickening perfume, that hung in the stairwell whenever she went out or came in?

Convinced I was being stalked by chemicals, I rang Jean to ask for an emergency appointment. Sitting in her office that afternoon, I tried to describe the building site my street had become, but was so overwhelmed by a sense of hopelessness that I broke down in tears.

"We must test you for building materials," said Jean, sympathetically. "Why don't you come to Greece with us in September? Dr. Rae and I are starting a conference center there, and I'll be taking a group of ten patients. It would do you good to get away, and the air there would be so much cleaner."

Not in Athens, it wouldn't be, I wanted to say, recalling my last visit there. Why was escape the only solution anyone had to offer? At best it could provide only temporary relief.

Persuaded that chemicals would pursue me even to the Aegean, I declined Jean's offer and drove home, more discouraged than ever. As I was parking my car, I saw a huge truck marked "Hydrochloric Acid" in front of the building next door. In the entrance hall, I encountered a new chemical odor. Seeing the caretaker there, I asked him what it was.

"It's probably coming from the penthouse," he said. "They had their carpets cleaned yesterday, and I guess that's what you smell."

At the clinic the next day, I was tested for dry rot, diesel fuel, soft woods, cement, and tobacco, with strong reactions to all. Arriving home, I saw workmen shoveling what looked like sand into the basement flat of Number 9. How many toxins had I inhaled from that renovation alone, I wondered—from the formaldehyde foam insulation in the walls they were knocking through, from the dust in the ripped-up floorboards, and from all the other detritus that was finding its way into my flat?

Spotting Ron, the works manager, standing outside, I asked him, "Ron, when did the demolition work begin on your site?"

"We started on January 16," he said.

Six months of pollution, then, from his building, and three months from the one on the other side.

Two days later, I detected a familiar odor in the entrance hall. Finding Ron there with a workman, I asked, "Do you know what the odor is here in the hall, Ron?"

"What odor?" he asked.

"You mean you can't smell it? It's the same as the one that comes through that hole in the wall outside my flat."

"Oh, that," he said. "It must be the Cuprinol we've been putting on the timber for the door frames next door."

"We don't smell it, you see," explained the workman, "because we work with it all day long."

But that's why it's so dangerous! I wanted to say. Instead, I said, "You know, you really should wear protective masks when working with such strong chemicals."

"Come to think of it," said Ron, "I've had a headache for several weeks. I wonder if that could be the reason."

"Well, the stuff must be safe," said the workman. "If it wasn't, we'd have been told to wear masks, or been given protective gloves, or something, wouldn't we?"

Two months later, I learned that Ron had been diagnosed with cancer.

INVISIBLE ENEMY

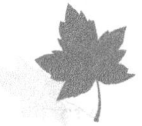

CHAPTER TEN

Thanks to the antigens for building materials, my symptoms eased over the summer. By September, however, my legs were aching and my heart was acting skittish again. More worrying were the two broken toes on my right foot, which hurt when I had to wear proper shoes. I also had a bunion to contend with.

Clearly, something had to be done, so my new GP sent me to see a foot surgeon, Mr. Baer. I dreaded the thought of another operation—not because I feared surgery, but because the anesthetic would be adding more chemicals to my overloaded system. Still, if I wanted to remain ambulatory, I had no choice.

Mr. Baer was a blunter version of the austere Dr. Thorne, with eyes that looked as though they had never smiled and a manner that forestalled all but the most determined question. He examined my toes and described the procedure he would perform.

"Now, I shall insert a steel pin in your big toe to keep it straight while it heals and in the other two toes…."

"Oh, I'm afraid I can't have the pin, Mr. Baer," I broke in. "You see, I'm chemically sensitive and my body won't tolerate a foreign substance."

"Nonsense," he said. "You cannot possibly be allergic to the pin. It's stainless steel, which is inert. It's all in your mind."

I drew a deep breath. "Why would my mind want to make my body suffer?" I asked. He gave me a sour look. I described for him my experience with the silicone breast implant, but I might have been explaining metaphysics to a butcher.

"If you refuse to have the pin," Baer said, "I cannot be responsible for the outcome. Furthermore," he warned, "if you don't have the pin, you will have to wear a cast for at least four weeks to keep your toes immobilized."

"Fine," I said. "I'll be happy to."

This knocked him off his perch for a moment, but he rallied and his manner hardened. Had I been more perceptive, I would have sensed the enmity our exchange had aroused, but I assumed he was just one more doctor for whom environmental illness was a female delusion.

As I surfaced from the anesthetic I could not believe the pain that was throbbing in my toes. How could such tiny bones cause such monumental agony? Painkillers offered some relief, but when I begged the nurse for more she refused. "You've been given the maximum dose allowed," she said. So I spent the sleepless night rocking and moaning in my hospital bed.

The next day I went home with a knee-high cast and a pair of crutches to which I quickly adapted. Had it not been for the kindness of my upstairs neighbor, however—a fellow American who saw me in the hall with my sticks one day and offered to do my grocery shopping when she did hers—the mechanics of living would have been a good deal more complicated than they were.

I was managing quite well when, days later, I felt my foot begin to swell inside the cast. Suspecting the nylon sutures, I made an appointment with Mr. Baer to have them taken out.

"Absolutely not," he replied. "The sutures must stay in or your toes won't heal properly."

"I understand that, Mr. Baer, but my foot is swelling and I know I'm reacting to the nylon."

"I have told you that nylon is inert," he said, in his

how-dare-you-know-more-about-your-body-than-I-do voice. "You cannot possibly be affected by the sutures."

I did not like Mr. Baer.

"Please," I begged. "Can't I persuade you to take them out?"

"No."

This threw me into confusion. I knew I was right, yet I was so ashamed of my freakish body, and so intimidated by Baer, I was afraid to stand up to the man. Within hours of returning home, however, my foot was screaming, "Get these things out of my toes!"

Two days later the swelling had reached my ankle. The next morning, it had spread to my calf and was pressing against the cast. Emboldened by fear, I went to see Baer again, determined this time to *make* him remove the sutures.

"After all," I pointed out, "the cast will be coming off in another week."

"Under no circumstance will I remove the cast *or* the sutures," he said, as if I had asked him to remove his clothes.

"But I can't bear the pressure, Mr. Baer. Please, *please*, take them out!" I begged.

"I'm warning you," he said. "If I remove the sutures before time, you will have to remain on crutches for another two weeks."

"I don't care," I cried. "Just take them out now!"

He studied me for a moment with something akin to contempt. Then he picked up the phone, rang the Brompton Hospital, and booked an appointment for the following day.

At the Brompton, I was shown to a cubicle off an open ward where I was told to wait for the surgeon. He arrived accompanied by a young assistant and after a perfunctory greeting, instructed me to lie down on the table. While Baer washed his hands and the assistant arranged some instruments on a tray, I studied the pattern in the curtain he had drawn to screen us from the communal room beyond.

Selecting a tool from the tray, Baer began to cut through the cast, while I waited, wondering what he would say when he saw my swollen calf. I heard him work his way through the plaster, felt the pieces fall away from my foot, and saw him hand them to his acolyte, but from Baer there came not a word. Instead, he began ripping out the stitches with such force I felt my toes were being raped. Screaming with pain, I tried to slide off the table, but the assistant's strong arms held me down. Mortified that my screams could be heard throughout the ward, I begged Baer to stop, but he went on pulling and tearing, like a butcher trussing a slab of meat on a chopping block. I so hated him in that moment I wished him violently dead! How gladly I would have driven a stake through his heart, if he'd had one. By the time he had finished, I was so shaken I could hardly speak.

"Why didn't you stop when I begged you to?" I demanded.

He gave me a thin token smile, like a modern Mengele. *"Well?"* I said.

"Well," he replied, "you said you didn't want an anesthetic."

"You *know* I didn't mean a *local* one!" I shot back. "You might at least have stopped when you saw I was in pain."

But he turned to his assistant, consigned the cast-making job to him and said goodbye, leaving me lying on the table trembling with fury and limp with shock.

The next morning the swelling was gone, and with it my rage of the day before. I was too glad the sutures were out to waste my energy cursing Baer and his butchery.

Five days later, however, my foot began to swell again. How could this be? The sutures were gone, and it couldn't be the plaster cast. Unwilling to confront the surgeon, I went to the Brompton Hospital's emergency room, prepared to tough it out with Baer on the phone, if necessary.

"I'm sorry," said the young doctor on duty, "but I'm not allowed to remove the cast or sutures without the consent of your surgeon. If you wish, I can ring him to ask his permission."

He returned to say that Baer was in the operating theater that morning and would not be in his office until after lunch. "I've left a message for him to ring me here, but it could be several hours before he returns the call. Do you want to wait?"

"All day if necessary," I replied.

For three hours, I sat in the large waiting room, watching the walking wounded come and go, while worrying about my foot and trying to finish *The Tibetan Book of the Dead*. At length, seeing the doctor heading toward me, I knew that a verdict was at hand.

"Mr. Baer has given his consent for the cast to be removed," he announced.

I could have hugged him for joy! Either Baer was thoroughly sick of me, I reckoned, or he no longer gave a damn. Or both.

The doctor proceeded to remove the cast, carefully unwinding the bloody gauze from around my toes. As he lifted the last piece, he paused, peered at my foot and said, "Hello, there's a suture here in one toe. Would you like me to take it out?"

"Yes, please," I said, stifling a cheer.

Had Baer overlooked the suture during his assault, I wondered, or had he left it there on purpose to prove a point? Would he have mentioned it if *he* had been the one to remove the cast? I neither knew nor cared, for by that evening the swelling had begun to go down.

So what if my toes didn't heal as perfectly as they would have done with the pins? I thought, stalking about on my sticks for another fortnight. At least my funny old body had proved that inert matter can be very *"ert"* indeed.

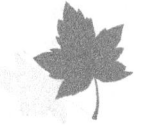

CHAPTER ELEVEN

Stuck as I was on a plateau with symptoms that had returned and antigens that no longer worked, I received Jean's approval in December to go to Dallas. Perhaps in Dr. Rae's environmentally controlled unit, I could find some of the answers that had eluded me in London.

Dr. Rae greeted me cordially, read my note from Jean, and ordered blood to be drawn for a round of tests. I was then driven with another patient to the ECU, which occupied one floor of a hospital twenty minutes away.

Before entering the unit, we passed through an antechamber where we relinquished our personal effects and exchanged our clothes for the white cotton scrubs that would be our uniform for the next two weeks. The door to the unit was as thick as a bank vault's and bore the familiar sign forbidding entry to anyone wearing perfume, makeup, hair spray, or shaving lotion.

Once admitted, we found ourselves in an antiseptic world of tiled floors, stainless steel walls, and chemical-free furnishings that were sparse, but serviceable. Vents in the ceiling delivered a steady flow of filtered air, their constant hum adding to the sense of being on a spaceship floating through the cosmos.

The only writing materials permitted were a lead pencil and a stenographer's pad; the only books those old enough to have lost the smell of print, but not yet old enough to have acquired the scent of mold. Taped to the wall above the scale on which we weighed ourselves each morning was a large square of aluminum foil, into which a patient had laboriously punched out the words:

> We are all faced with brilliant opportunities, brilliantly disguised as insurmountable problems.

Each evening, Dr. Rae arrived to make his rounds, accompanied by young Dr. Evans, who was on duty during the day. In the testing room a lone nurse was doing her best to cope with twenty-six patients. There should have been three nurses on duty, but because of the Christmas holiday the unit was short-staffed.

Patients were having familiar reactions to the antigens. One woman grew tearful when testing for orrisroot—a component of perfume, hair spray, and shaving cream. Another grew hyperactive, and a third grew sleepy, while others, challenged with the same substance, became irascible or depressed.

Two women wore charcoal masks even in the unit.

"We're affected by the electronic equipment at the nurses' station," one of them explained.

No wonder doctors thought our problems had more to do with our minds than our molecules, but my heart went out to them—and to every sufferer I met in the ECU, most of whom had immune systems far more damaged than mine.

And yet, I began to question the long-term validity of the antigen approach, for even after weeks of testing some patients still could not tolerate more than a few foods. Surely, the body needed a variety of nutrients to heal.

Discussing my symptoms with Dr. Evans one day, I described the feeling of an acid creeping under my scalp.

"I know," he nodded. "It's like a headache."

"It is not in the least like a headache," I said, bristling at the glib reply. Good grief, I thought; if a clinical ecology doctor can't be curious, what am I doing here?

"It's just that—it's such a peculiar symptom," he said, lamely, as though that absolved him of the need to discover its cause.

"Of course it's peculiar," I said. "We're all peculiar here."

"Well," he hedged, backing away from the problem and toward the door, "let's see how you get on with the double-blind chemical tests and the fast."

The chemical booth formed part of a small area that included a changing room, a shower, and a heart-monitoring machine. Although some of the tests would involve a placebo, the shower and shampoo were obligatory after each one. I exchanged my scrub suit for a cotton kimono and entered the chamber. A young technician, Debbie, took my blood pressure, gave me a pulmonary test, and attached electrodes to my chest and legs.

"You're to take your pulse three times during the ten-minute test," said Debbie, showing me how. "Then give me the reading and report any symptoms you may have."

She placed a canister on the floor, instructing me to unscrew the cap of the unlabeled bottle inside after she left. "The bottle contains either a placebo or a chemical, which you will breathe for a certain period of time," she explained.

She closed the hermetically sealed door and took up her post by the table outside with the monitoring equipment. A window in the door allowed her to observe my reactions, while we communicated through an intercom.

There were six tests in all. At the end of each I was to return to my room and record my pulse rate at fifteen-minute intervals for an hour, together with any symptoms. I had no reaction to the contents of the first bottle, which I assumed was a placebo. The second one released an odor that smelled like nail varnish or fresh paint. My nose clogged up, I felt dizzy and began to sneeze. The third test was also a placebo, but the contents of the fourth bottle made me feel light-headed, and I was aware of being garrulous with Debbie.

When I returned to my room, I developed a slight tremor in my hands, which spread to my thighs and ended in a mild panic attack. By the time Debbie arrived two hours later, the symptoms were gone.

"I could tell you were hyper on that last test," she said, "because you became very loquacious, and you're not normally the chatty type. You seem to be calmer within yourself than most of the people we see here."

"What was the chemical?" I asked, eagerly.

"Sorry," she said, "I'm not allowed to say."

Later, I learned it was formaldehyde.

Environmentally ill patients know from experience that low-grade, long-term toxicity can result in a hyper-acute sense of taste, hearing, or smell. The smallest whiff of fragrance in the ECU's purified air was like an assault on my hyperactive hippocampus. Twice, I suspected a nurse of using perfume, which was forbidden in the unit. In each case, it turned out the nurse in question had washed her hair the night before, and it was the trace of phthalates in her shampoo rinse that had triggered my twitchy olfactory nerves. Hard though it was to live with such exaggerated acuity, it did at least warn me of the things I needed to avoid.

Dr. Rae stressed this point on one of his visits when he advised us not to go into public places for several weeks after we left the unit.

"You will be extremely vulnerable for a while," he warned. "Inhalants such as phenol, formaldehyde, and tobacco smoke are pervasive in enclosed areas. No malls, drugstores, or department stores. The rule is: If you can smell it, avoid it."

I was reminded of the obstacle course I had to run each time I went to Harrods, to avoid being sprayed with scent by a roaming predator from the perfume counter.

On December 20, the four-day fast began. I weighed 121 pounds and couldn't wait to begin. What I resented most about my condition was that it forced me to think about food fourteen hours a day. The fast, therefore, would be a relief.

At the end of the first day I felt weak and my brain was muddled. The second day I rallied, but on the third, I woke with a headache. Dr. Evans came by to tell me that the chemical tests showed my allergies were primarily chemical, which I already knew. By the fourth day I had lost eight pounds, my symptoms had vanished, and I felt I could levitate.

Christmas Day dawned bleak and beautiful, the whitewashed world beyond my window as surreal as the one in which I was temporarily cocooned. The twenty-fifth also marked the end of the fast and the beginning of single-food meals. Patients could choose the one food they would eat each day, so I chose a baked apple. I had consumed only half when my scalp woke up, my hands turned red, and my heart began to do its funny jig.

The had the same reaction each day, no matter what food I chose. I recalled Randolph telling me about patients whose symptoms vanished after a five-day fast, only to return when a drop of an allergen was placed under their tongue. It what way, then, could fasting either help or cure?

It didn't help that the food was badly cooked and kept in warming compartments until mealtime. When patients complained about the half-cooked rice swimming in a bowl of glutinous liquid, we were told it was because a temporary staff was on duty over Christmas.

When Dr. Rae came by the next day, I described for him the return of my symptoms when I introduced single-food meals.

"I'm sure it's just an allergy that will clear up if you stay on the rotation diet," he said.

At the mention of the "rotation diet" my heart sank. I had tried that diet the year before and had given up after six months—not because it didn't help, but because it was so time-consuming.

The idea was to eat the widest variety of foods in order to control existing allergies and prevent the formation of new ones. Since the transit time through the human digestive system requires up to three days, no single food can be repeated within four days—a tricky challenge if one is a vegetarian. It became even trickier when I found that certain vegetables belong to the same family—not just logical ones, such as cauliflower, broccoli, and sprouts, but peculiar ones, like potato, eggplant, and tomato. This meant that I had to avoid *every* family member for four days.

Sticking a chart of these ancestral trees on my kitchen wall, I was dismayed to discover how many of my favorite vegetables belonged to the same clan. The diet was a gastronomic seat belt—safe, but restricting—and because foods had to be eaten in a certain order, they needed to be prepared in advance and stored in the freezer.

The thought of having to do all that cooking, wrapping, dating, and storing again was too depressing to contemplate. When, oh when, would I have time to *write*?

"Meanwhile," said Dr. Rae, "I think you should leave London and go live somewhere by the sea."

Oh no! I thought. Had I come all this way and spent all this money, only to receive from Rae the same advice Clive had been giving me for free?

The day I left the ECU I was more sensitive than when I went in. As I stepped into the corridor, the hospital's odors knocked me sideways. I had forgotten how dangerous the outside world could be, with its perfume and pollution and noise, so the shock of reentry was seismic. I paid my bill as fast as I could and rushed from the building, gasping for air. Was I doomed to spend the rest of my life in this pan-reactive state? I thought of other, smaller animal species, whose very survival depends on their delicate sense of smell. Are we destroying *their* early warning system, as well as our own, by the toxic environment we are creating? When we can no longer see, hear, smell, or sense the enemy, it is already within the gates.

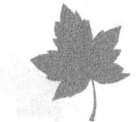

CHAPTER TWELVE

Before leaving the ECU, I asked Dr. Rae if he knew a dentist he could recommend. An automobile accident in 1952 had left me with a broken jaw, some missing teeth, and a nasty scar on my chin. A brilliant dentist in Beverly Hills had designed a partial that served me well for twenty-five years. Now, however, due to the normal changes that occur in the mouth, it needed to be redone. Newly aware of the perils in dentistry for the chemically sensitive, I was afraid to risk an orthodox dentist in London.

"I know an excellent dentist," Rae said, "but you must warn him not to use epinephrine in the anesthetic." Wouldn't he know that if he has treated patients with environmental illness, I thought? "Epinephrine provides the staying power," Rae explained, "so without it, you'll need more frequent injections. If you decide to have the work done here, a patient of mine has a 'safe house' where you can stay as a paying guest. Let me know and I'll find out if Willie Mae has an available room."

Willie Mae Phipps was a widow in her early seventies: pink hairnet, beige cardigan flung over a flowered house dress, white ankle socks, and the kind of Texas drawl that did funny things to her vowels. An ardent Baptist, she kept her kitchen radio tuned permanently to one of the many religious stations in Dallas, which provided a gospel-thumping backdrop to mealtime conversations. Pictures of angels in various attitudes of prayer adorned her walls, with pride of place held by a large plate inscribed with The Lord's Prayer that hung next to the kitchen table.

As I had only the sketchiest knowledge about the Baptist faith, I asked Willie Mae about its tenets one day when we were in the kitchen.

"You gotta be saved," she said, chucking potato skins into the compost basket. "If you don't accept Jesus Christ as your Lord, you can't be saved. When you die, you'll be judged and sent straight down to Hell."

Hell or no, Willie Mae offered refuge to those for whom the chemical products in the average hotel would have been akin to purgatory. When I arrived in January, I found another patient, Louise, already installed. Thin, pale, and on the cusp of forty, Louise had been an administrative official at a school when someone emptied cleaning fluid down the drain of a supply room across the hall from her office. Without knowing why, she became ill and disoriented, and her body went into spasms.

"No one knew what was wrong with me," she said. "I fell into a coma and went blind for a while. Months later, when I recovered enough to return to work, I was exposed to another chemical accident. This time, my immune system was virtually destroyed. If I held a telephone receiver against my ear, I felt sharp pains shooting through my head. The doctors thought I was loopy, of course, but when I had the mercury amalgam fillings removed from my teeth, that particular symptom disappeared."

After twenty days of antigen testing, Louise could eat only nine foods without having a severe allergic reaction, although she should have been able to eat a minimum of sixteen. Odors that I could tolerate wiped her out, especially those that abound in public places. If she had to enter a store or fly in a plane, she wore a grotesque charcoal mask that made her look like a deep-sea diver or an alien from outer space. Even my "unscented" face powder bothered her, so I refrained from using it while there.

"The reason I sleep here in the kitchen on a folding bed is because I couldn't tolerate the mold in that upstairs bedroom," Louise explained, referring to the room I had just inherited. "It's truly awful."

Mold wasn't the half of it. The rectangular room had a bed at one end and at the other, a stack of velour-covered chairs that looked as though they had been stored there for years. Two sheet-covered boxes lined one wall, while standing against the opposite wall was a portable clothes rack, its vintage garments lightly mantled with dust.

Had Rae ever vetted Willie Mae's house, I wondered, or had he taken her word for it that it was safe? It may have been safe for her, but what is safe for one sensitive patient can be fraught with danger for another. At least I could do something about those tumbleweeds of dust under the bed.

My first night in the room, the thermometer fell to 20 degrees Fahrenheit and the electric heater was broken.

"You'll have to pay extra for heat," said Willie Mae the next morning, when I mentioned the cold. It took three days for the heater to be repaired. Meanwhile, whether because of the mold, the dust, or the perishing cold, my rhinitis grew steadily worse.

On January 6, I met with Dr. Rae to discuss the chemical analysis of the two blood samples that were taken the day I arrived.

"One shows moderate levels of pentylphenol and chloroprene in the serum," he said, reading from the report, "as well as styrene and benzene."

"What does pentylphenol do?" I asked. "It doesn't sound body-friendly."

"It's used in treating wood and leathers, things such as shoes and handbags."

"And where would I have picked up the styrene?"

"That would have come from breathing fumes given off by packing materials, or from drinking out of styrene cups, hot liquids especially."

"Which I never do."

"Of greater concern, though," said Rae, "is the test for volatiles, which shows a high amount of methylene chloride."

"That sounds ominous. Where would that have come from?"

"From inhaling the propellant in aerosol cans, for instance, such as those used for pesticides." Oh, no, that insect-killer again! "Of course," Rae added, "you would have been more susceptible to methylene chloride if you had other chemicals in your body, which you do. What makes it more worrisome is that you wear contact lenses."

"Why contact lenses?" I asked, surprised.

"Because they absorb strong vapors and hold them against your eyes, which can cause irritation or damage. The worst problem with methylene chloride, however, is the way it combines with hemoglobin in the blood to create carbon monoxide. This prevents the blood from carrying oxygen to the tissues."

More chemicals to worry about then, and still no way to get them out of my system.

A week had gone by before I realized that the supplements I should have been taking during that time hadn't arrived, and neither had the results of my other tests. When I rang Rae's office to inquire, I learned they had been sent to London. No one had informed them I would be staying on for a month. By the time I returned home, I had missed four weeks of supplements that might or might not have forestalled the ongoing collapse of my immune system.

On the seventh I met Dr. Benson, the dentist Rae recommended. A likable, soft-spoken man, he examined my partial and assured me he could replicate it. After taking X-rays he found decay under two teeth, as well as mercury amalgam under two fillings.

"To remove the amalgam and deal with the decay, I will have to redo the precision inlays on both sides," he said. "I'm also concerned about a root canal on the lower left side, because formaldehyde is usually poured into the root to numb the nerve. This continues to leach into the gums and really should be removed."

This was a bad surprise; I hadn't anticipated such extensive dental work. Dr. Benson gave me an appointment for the tenth, and I returned to Willie Mae's in time to see a large oxygen tank being delivered to the house.

"It's for Betty," she said, "the patient who's arriving tonight from New Jersey. She's extremely sensitive and always stays with me when she comes here for treatment with Dr. Rae."

I heard Betty's arrival downstairs at half past ten that night, but didn't meet her until lunch the next day. A lively brunette in her forties, she, too, had suffered a series of chemical accidents that virtually destroyed her immune system.

"After working in an aircraft assembly plant for several years," she said, in answer to my question, "I was so affected by the chemicals that I left and found a job in what I thought was the safer environment of an office. Unfortunately, they had installed new carpeting, and the out-gassing chemicals from the carpet and underlay were even worse." The final blow had been an accident at work, similar to the one Louise had suffered. "It's left me hypersensitive to certain foods," Betty explained, "which is why I need to have oxygen nearby in case of an emergency."

Minutes later, she suddenly dropped her fork, pointed to the mashed potatoes on her plate and gasped, "Is there butter in this?"

"Only a smidgen," said Willie Mae, alarmed.

"I've got to have oxygen!" cried Betty, stumbling from the table and running to her room.

"I forgot she can't tolerate butter," said Willie Mae, looking stricken.

While Betty was absent the three of us sat in worried silence, moving the food around on our plates, our minds troubled, our appetites gone. My own thoughts turned to the nature of suffering and something I'd read by Edith Hamilton in *The Greek Way:*

Pain is the most individualizing thing on earth…. To suffer is to be alone. To watch another suffer is to know the barrier that shuts each of us away by himself.

When Betty returned, she showed us her swollen fingers and the palms of her hands, which were now rough and cracked.

"This is what happens when I'm having a reaction," she explained. "If I eat anything with butter in it, my whole body goes haywire. My fingers swell up and I become incoherent and act like a crazy woman. Ten minutes on my oxygen tank with a shot of serotonin, and I'm almost normal again."

How diverse, I thought, are the stigmata of allergy.

I was feeling the need for some exercise the next day, so—forgetting Rae's warning about public places—I decided to go to a nearby mall and look for some walking shoes. Scarcely had I entered the building, when the onslaught of odors in the concourse had me reeling. *Panic stations!* cried my body. I bought the first comfortable pair of shoes I could find and fled the mall with them on.

On the walk back to Willie Mae's, I was pleased to discover that my emergency purchase was so comfortable. After a while, however, I felt a mild burning in the insteps. As soon as I reached the house, I took off the shoes and the burning stopped, but when I wore them the next day it returned.

I was describing this oddity at dinner that evening, when Betty said, "Let me see the shoes."

"Oh, they're all leather," I assured her, as I went to fetch one.

Betty held the shoe in one hand and felt around inside with the other.

"It may be leather on the outside," she said, handing it back to me, "but the interlining feels like acrylic. I'll bet that's what's affecting you—that, and your nylon stockings."

So eager had I been to escape the mall, I hadn't noticed the shiny mesh lining inside—nor would I have questioned it if I had, for it covered the soft padding that made the shoes so comfortable.

"The reason I spotted it," explained Betty, "is because once, when I bought a new cotton dress, I couldn't understand why it bothered me each time I wore it. Eventually, suspecting the nylon label in the back, I cut it out, and after that, the dress was fine. So I removed the labels from all my clothes."

"That's why people think we're crazy," said Louise, who knew from long experience. "They don't understand that when the immune system collapses, virtually anything can affect you, no matter how crazy it seems."

"The trouble is," said Willie Mae, "most doctors don't know any more about how chemicals affect the body than we do ourselves."

"That's right," said Betty. "Environmental illness has made sleuths of us all. We have to be our own detectives, because doctors don't have time to track down the cause of each patient's problem, and even if they did, few would want to." Turning again to me, she said, "It doesn't look as though that lining stuff can be removed from your shoes, but if you wear dark cotton socks, they should protect you."

When I told Dr. Rae about the acrylic the next day, he seemed surprised.

"It's the first time I've heard of such a peculiar sensitivity," he said.

"Surely not," I replied. "I've seen far stranger reactions in the testing room."

But then, Rae could hardly have been expected to know every queer symptom that turned up at his clinic. At least he was trying to help those who had exhausted everything conventional medicine had to offer.

In the end, it was not from the doctors in Dallas that I learned the most; it was from Betty and Louise, and from all the chemically damaged patients I met in the ECU.

And it was Betty, a few days later, who gave me advice that may even have saved my life.

CHAPTER THIRTEEN

On January 10, Dr. Benson began to drill out the old inlays before tackling the amalgam and decay that lay underneath. "I think you're doing quite well without the epinephrine," he said. The next day's session went almost as well, although I needed more injections of the anesthetic. By the third session, however, I was feeling distinctly fragile. Even before Benson had finished, my heart was fibrillating and my head felt as though it was filled with helium.

"Well, that's it," said Benson, rolling his stool away from the chair. "We're done. I must say, you've held up better than I expected."

He retreated to the counter behind me and began to prepare the alginate for the impression tray. Relieved the worst was over, I closed my eyes and breathed deeply, letting the coils of nervous tension begin to unwind. As my mind drifted into a hypnagogic state, amorphous images rose and dissolved behind my closed eyelids. I seemed to be floating in another dimension—light-headed, bodiless, and blissfully free.

Suddenly my heart lurched, my blood sugar dropped, and I felt the life force drain from my being. *I'm dying*, I thought. I tried to speak, but no sound came. I tried to move, but the link between brain and body had been cut.

Dr. Benson reappeared and began to ease the impression tray into my mouth. Even in my parlous state I could see the irony of having a mold made of my teeth just as the rest of me was about to expire. By the time he removed the tray, however, I had been granted a reprieve.

While Benson returned to the counter to prepare the cement for the temporary caps, I struggled to clear the fog from my brain. At length, I regained my voice and was able to ask, "Dr. Benson ... when you were preparing the alginate ... did you introduce a new substance into the room?"

"No, nothing that wasn't out before. Why?"

"Because I felt as though I...." But the fog closed in again and I grew confused. "Oh, nothing."

My mouth felt dry. I thought of the bottle of mineral water in my bag and tried to rise, but my legs had turned to jelly. Benson returned, and by the time he'd cemented the caps, I had recovered enough to tell him what happened.

"Well, you have had a lot of anesthetic today," he said.

At the end of the session I still felt too physically shaken to drive home safely, so I decided to wait in the reception room until my head cleared. But shouldn't Benson have suggested this? For a dentist with experience of chemically sensitive patients, he seemed surprisingly clueless about the basic precautions.

At dinner that evening, I was describing my near-death experience in the dental chair, when Betty cut in, her eyes wide with concern.

"You mean you weren't wearing an oxygen mask while he worked on you?"

"No, should I have been?"

"Of course! Sensitive patients should never have dental work done without oxygen. I'm surprised he didn't insist on it himself."

"I don't think he knew," I said, feeling stupid—and then alarmed.

"Well, frankly," said Betty, "I think you've had far too much work done on your teeth so soon after leaving the unit. Your immune system is too vulnerable to have had that much anesthetic, even without the epinephrine. Why, do you realize," she added, addressing the table, "that all of us here on this planet are living with one-third less oxygen than was originally here? One-third less than we should be breathing right now!"

"That wouldn't surprise me," said Louise, "the way we've been cutting down forests and spreading chemicals everywhere." Willie Mae nodded her agreement.

"Imagine how we would feel if we lived in a world without chemicals and had a third more oxygen to breathe," Betty went on. "Why, we would be amazed at our sense of well-being!"

Suddenly, our attention was drawn to a news item on the radio, which had been chattering away in the background: *A plant near a major city in Texas will soon be manufacturing methyl isocyanate.*

"Isn't that the chemical that devastated Bhopal in India?" I said, the memory of that horror still etched on my mind.

A silence fell as we listened to the rest of the report, exchanging glances and shaking our heads. Scarcely a week went by without news of a chemical accident somewhere—a truck shedding its toxic load on a highway or a tanker spilling its oil into the sea—accidents followed invariably by official assurances that "There is no immediate danger."

After a recent chemical spill in California, motorists were told, "No one having temporary breathing or eye difficulties will experience any lasting damage." How did they know? It could be years before the effects of that exposure became known, by which time the cause would have been forgotten and it would be too late to sue; too late, also, for the damage to be undone.

When the report ended, Betty rose and took her plate to the sink. Returning to the table, she stood with her hand on her hip and said, "Do you know what the most endangered species on this planet *really is*? It's us. We're the canaries keeling over to warn of the dangers ahead if we keep fouling our nest the way we're doing."

"The trouble is," said Louise, her sad eyes looking sadder, "no one is listening. Besides, who will protect us from the pharmaceutical companies? Not the FDA—not when Big Pharma pours millions of dollars into the coffers of both parties."

"That's right," said Willie Mae. "Most people never suspect their aches and pains, like arthritis, could be caused by chemicals, so they make things worse by taking drugs. And the doctors don't tell them, 'cause they don't know themselves."

"And most people don't even care," I said.

"I'll tell you something else," said Betty, her voice crisp with contempt. "We take better care of our cars than we do of our bodies!"

Later that evening, while helping Willie Mae with the dishes, I noticed that whenever I touched something metal, like a saucepan, I experienced an odd metallic taste on my tongue. That night, before going to bed, I peered into the back of my mouth with a pocket mirror. As I had feared, the caps Benson had put on my teeth were metal.

Aware of the galvanic reaction mixed metals create in the mouth, I suspected they were interacting with a couple of gold inlays. Had I not been so distracted by imminent death during that last session, I might have noticed what Benson was doing and could have stopped him.

I was on the phone the moment his office opened the next morning.

"Dr. Benson, the caps you put on my teeth yesterday … what are they made of?"

"They're aluminum."

"Aluminum!" I cried. How could anyone with the least knowledge of chemical sensitivity have put aluminum in my mouth? "Well, I think I'm reacting to the metal."

Hearing the alarm in my voice, he said, "If you want to come in this morning I can change them to stainless steel for you."

I jumped into my rented hatchback and sped to his office—passing a giant billboard sign that said "JESUS ALONE IS THE ANSWER!"

Not when you need a good dentist.

"I've never had a patient who was allergic to aluminum before," said Benson, as he replaced the offending caps, "but then I don't know much about allergies."

It was too late to wonder why Rae had recommended him or why I had let him finish the job, when my body had been warning me for days. I drove back to Willie Mae's with a new sense of foreboding.

That night, I came down with the flu.

For my penultimate dental appointment, I was wearing an oxygen mask, thanks to Betty's hectoring. The difference it made was dramatic. Without the oxygen I might well have come to grief, for Benson was finding it harder this time to keep me desensitized.

"I don't know why you're metabolizing more quickly today than you did before," he said.

"I do. It's because I'm full of chemicals, that's why."

"Oh, is that it?"

He presented the new partial and my apprehension grew. It did not look like the original. Benson eased it into my mouth and I tested the fit with my fingers.

"It doesn't feel as secure as the old one," I said.

"It just needs a bit of adjusting," he replied, with more confidence than I felt able to share. He removed the partial and worked on it for a few minutes, before positioning it again in my mouth.

"It still doesn't feel right," I said, with mounting concern.

"Well, it may take a few days for your teeth to adjust to it," said Benson.

Too late I knew it had been a costly disaster, and would have to be redone when I returned to London—that is, if I could find a dentist there willing and able to undo the damage Benson had done. Beguiled by the man's niceness, I now felt betrayed by his ineptitude. Not only had he ruined my mouth, his ignorance had almost cost me my life.

"Good grief!" exclaimed Betty when I came in the door. "You look like the stuffing's been knocked out of you, girl. Didn't he give you any oxygen?" I shook my head yes. "Well, then, you need some more. Come with me!" She marched me into her room and hooked me up to her oxygen cylinder. "Now you stay there until you're fully recovered, do you hear?"

I felt far safer in Betty's hands than I did in those of the dentist. Within a short time my strength had returned, and I joined Betty in the kitchen, in time to give her a hand with dinner and a grateful hug.

The final session nearly did me in, oxygen notwithstanding. Each time Benson cemented a tooth, the nerve spasmed and my body shrieked *No more anesthetic!* I managed to get through the last 30 minutes without it, but had it not been for Betty's benevolent bullying, my story might have ended in Dallas.

"How did he get it so wrong?" I wailed to her that evening. "All he had to do was copy the original, which he had right there in front of his nose for weeks!"

After my return to London, I found a wonderful dentist who, if he couldn't correct Benson's worst mistakes, he at least managed to transform a dental disaster into something I've been able to live with.

Two years later, I received a letter from Louise, telling me she'd heard the ECU had been closed after a patient there had died while having some dental work done.

Sadly, the news came too late to share with Betty. Word of her death reached me a year after I returned to England.

CHAPTER FOURTEEN

I flew home from Dallas wearing a charcoal mask for most of the journey to filter the cabin's recycled air. When I opened the front door I was greeted by the smell of varnish in the entrance hall; a neighbor was having her parquet floor refinished. I turned on the central heating and thought I could smell the odorless gas. I couldn't, but in bed that night my heart skipped about erratically in my chest. *Why, oh why do these poisons pursue me?* I cried out to an indifferent God. God's sole reply was a new array of symptoms.

With a zeal known only to the terminally allergic, I set about transforming my flat from an ecological threat into a toxin-free oasis—learning in the process how hard it is, and how expensive, to rely on organic products alone.

After exchanging the few remaining chemical items under my sink for safer (and less efficient) substitutes, I replaced the carpeting in my bedroom with tile, the synthetic fabrics with cotton, and gave my new scarcely worn polyester caftan to Oxfam. As for the outside environment, however, I could do nothing.

Sifting through the mail that had arrived in my absence, I found the supplements and lab results that should have been sent to me in Dallas. The lab confirmed what I already knew.

Meanwhile, in addition to tachycardia, my brain had been going AWOL. I caught myself doing mindless things, such as throwing socks into the wastebasket instead of the laundry hamper and searching for my keys, which turned up in odd places instead of where they belonged.

Fear of dementia loomed large. As for God—if He happened to be listening, all I asked of Him was that He send me an answer soon—in *this* lifetime, if possible.

Adding to my discouragement that spring was the thought of all the food preparation I would have to do for the rotation diet. I wanted to *write,* damn it, not cook! All I asked of food was that it be fresh, organic, and uncontaminated.

In May, I had the gas boiler removed and the central heating changed from gas to electricity, a step recommended by Randolph and Rae. The pipes were capped on the eighth, and on the twelfth, I realized I hadn't had a tachycardia incident since. My hay fever, however, had returned with a vengeance. Either there was more pollen in the air that spring, or the antigens no longer worked.

Each time I went to the clinic for an intravenous drip, my veins went into hiding. When the nurse couldn't find a vein she would turn me over to Jean, whose expertise invariably found one on the first try. At the end of June, however, my veins shut down altogether, and when even Jean had trouble tapping a vein, I knew that clinical ecology had done as much for me as it could.

I had been having doubts about the vaccination approach—at least for me, notwithstanding its effectiveness for others. True, the antigens did neutralize the effects of harmful substances that could not be avoided, but to neutralize is not to cure. A body compromised by chemicals needs to be purged of them, not helped to withstand them, except as a temporary measure. For all its virtues, the vaccination method had no program for radical detoxification, and mainstream medicine did not even acknowledge the need for one. If homeopathy wasn't the answer—well, no one cure works for everyone. Where, then, I wondered, was the cure for me?

"You know," said Clive, on one of his visits that summer, "I may not be able to solve your problem after all. I've tried everything I can think of, but I'm afraid I've shot my bolt."

I had known for some time that neither Clive nor crystals could be the answer. Indeed, given my body's reaction to the stones, crystals were part of the problem. But I had become so addicted to our experiments, I didn't want them to end.

Much of what sustained me for six years had been the knowledge that Clive—practical, pragmatic, and profoundly leery of mysticism—could validate the source of my physical torment. He, too, could feel the same fractured energy line; he, too, could feel the polluted stream, only he needed a divining rod to find them.

If his efforts to neutralize these energies had failed, at least he had proved their telluric origin. Moreover, he had given me hope when I'd desperately needed something to cling to. And such is the nature of hope that even false hope can sustain us through trials that, without it, we might not be able to bear.

Two nights after Clive's visit, I found myself again in that familiar hell wherein sanity is destroyed, reason is absent, and consciousness splinters into a thousand fragments. Casting about for something to anchor my mind, I reached for the book on my bedside table. Its title was *A Time to Heal,* and its author, Beata Bishop, was a personal friend. The book describes her healing of malignant melanoma through an unconventional nutritional regime. That night, as my thinning carapace threatened once more to collapse, my friend's account of her triumph over cancer was just what I needed to get me through the long hours until dawn.

Beata's cancer began as a mole on her shin. When it became enlarged, her oncologist diagnosed it as melanoma and it was surgically removed. A painful skin graft followed, but the cancer returned within a year and had spread to her groin. Unwilling to submit to a second operation that offered only a poor chance of success, Beata decided to try the Gerson Therapy in Mexico, which was virtually unknown at the time.

I had followed her adventure, admiring her courage while blanching at the many strictures the therapy imposed. It did not merely advise reducing salt, sugar, coffee, wheat, meat, alcohol, tobacco, and dairy products—it *forbade* them. How, I wondered, could one endure a regime that banished from the table everything that made eating such a sensuous pleasure? How, for that matter, could cancer be cured by nutrition alone?

Yet Beata *was* cured—not only of stage four cancer, but also of frequent migraines, chronic dental abscesses, and diabetes. She had even been cured of her thirty-year addiction to nicotine. This had been a problem for us both when we shared a room at one of the weekend conferences we attended.

We had met at one such conference, sitting opposite each other at the vegetarian table for lunch, each feeling as though we had met before. We hadn't—I could not have met someone as sophisticated as Beata and forgotten her for an instant. Her faint accent, and the way she surveyed me with half-closed eyelids while blowing a stream of smoke toward the ceiling, set her apart from most of our fellow conferees. That day marked the start of our friendship, which was enhanced, for me, by Beata's knowledge of all the things I was so eager to learn.

By 1980, however, she was coping with cancer, while my struggle with chemicals had just begun. I don't think either of us fully appreciated what the other was going through at the time, since there were periods when we scarcely saw each other. As Beata later told me, "I often felt we existed in two different kinds of reality."

I suppose we did. Beata's reality was clear and focused, grounded in a lifetime of journalism and preparing for a practice in psychotherapy when she retired. My reality was vague and dreamy and wandering all over the place, which drove us both to distraction. Yet a curious bond developed between us, which I don't think either of us could have defined.

I opened Beata's book and read again the inscription she had written on the title page:

For Faye—whose path keeps crossing and touching
mine, with friendship and love,
—*Beata*

I began to read, torn between absorption in her story and envy of her narrative skill, for Beata was a wonderful writer. As a features writer for the BBC, she had already published two books. Reading about her struggle with cancer, however, I was struck by how differently we responded to events of a similar nature. It may even have been our differences that attracted us to each other.

Beata was a transplanted Hungarian, and a left-brain Gemini/Scorpio; quick-witted, impatient, and intellectual. I was a transplanted American, and a right-brain Scorpio/Cancer; slow-witted, absent-minded, and self-taught. Yet, as I read about the circumstance that led her to embark on such a radical journey, I sensed that her story might hold the key to my own darkening dilemma.

If so, it would not be the first time I had followed in Beata's footsteps. She had introduced me to the transpersonal psychology workshops, which I had enjoyed despite the no-show of that sage on the mountaintop. Looking back, I suspect the reason he didn't turn up was that he knew how unteachable I am by words alone. I seem to need a good kick in the backside to learn anything at all.

When I told Beata I had found my original birth certificate, with the names of my parents and the hour of my birth, she took me to one of the finest astrologers in England to have my chart read. Listening to the tape of that reading recently, I recalled my amusement when the astrologer said:

"Now, your chart shows a strong unconventional side; unusual, eccentric ... a bit way-out."

She could not have been more wrong, I thought. There were no conventions I wanted to flout, no rules I wished to defy. On the contrary, I mourned the loss of so many of the things I cherished that were quintessentially English, such as civility, good manners, tempered speech, a sly sense of humor, and a broad tolerance of eccentricity. Moreover, I viewed those who strive to be unconventional as merely absurd.

As I read Beata's story that night, I recalled a discussion we'd had once about my pesticide problem. She had suggested I try the Gerson Therapy, but I had dismissed the idea, reminding her that I had been cancer-free since 1974.

"That doesn't matter," she said. "The therapy is nonspecific—it's not just for cancer."

"Even so," I countered, "how could a vegan regime purge my body of the chemicals it has taken me a lifetime to acquire?"

"Because the therapy detoxifies the body and rebuilds the immune system," she explained, with infinite patience. "I see no reason why it shouldn't work for you as it has for me."

Detoxifies the body and rebuilds the immune system—the very things I knew I needed if my health was to be restored. Still, I doubted I could stick to such a demanding regime. Yet if not this, what then? I could not go on much longer as I was.

That night, as chemical demons closed in on me again, I decided that if Beata's footsteps were leading to Mexico, I would follow them even across the sea. But first, I needed to know more specifically what the therapy entailed.

I rang her the next day to say how much I was enjoying her book and to thank her for getting me through the night.

"Beata," I said, "I'm thinking of doing the Gerson Therapy. When can you come to lunch and give me the shove I need?"

CHAPTER FIFTEEN

She arrived looking wonderfully fit and full of energy, her mind as quick and incisive as ever, her tongue only occasionally sharp-edged. If proof of the therapy's success were needed, Beata could not have been bettered. We embraced, and after catching up on our separate lives, I got down to the purpose of our meeting.

"I don't know what to do about the chemicals in my system, Beata. I seem to be growing more sensitive to more things each day, and more discouraged. While reading your book last night, it came to me that as I've run out of options I might as well try the Gerson Therapy."

"Good!" she exclaimed, having gotten through to me at last. "I've felt for some time that a good detox with hyper-nutrition would be bound to improve your condition, if it doesn't cure it completely."

"What I find so off-putting, though, is the prospect of all those juices, not to mention the coffee enemas!"

She smiled. "They're really not bad at all. Anyway," she added, with a whiff of condescension, "as you don't have cancer, you probably won't be doing the full intensive therapy. I expect you will only have to do the modified diet, with fewer juices and enemas."

The mild put-down should not have rankled, but it did. Well I'd *had* cancer, dammit. I had even given a breast to the disease, which some might consider a worse disfigurement than a scar on the shin. But Beata was merely reflecting the universal view that cancer is the Queen Bee— or rather, the Queen C—of diseases; the one against which all toxic threats are measured, and the one that receives the most funding, with the poorest return on that investment.

Then too, like most people Beata had no idea what environmental illness entailed. With no lump or bump to display, no fearful label to intone, my problem inspired derision more often than sympathy.

"As for the vegetable juices," Beata was saying, "you'll need the kind of juicing machine that grinds the vegetables—not a centrifugal one—and also a separate press. The trouble with centrifugal juicers is that they produce an exchange of positive and negative electricity. That destroys the oxidizing enzymes needed to restore the immune system."

"But why so many juices?" I persisted. "Isn't it eight or ten a day?"

"Thirteen, actually, at the start."

"Thirteen! Doesn't the body rebel?"

"Not really. The reason for so many juices is that you have to bombard the depleted body at short and regular intervals with live vitamins, minerals, and oxidizing enzymes. It's only in juice form that you can ingest and absorb the huge amounts of nutrients needed."

"And the coffee enemas? Why coffee? It seems perverse to be putting it up your bottom while forbidding its more pleasurable consumption."

Beata laughed. "It has an altogether different effect when used at the other end," she explained. "The caffeine dilates the bile ducts, which allows the liver to release accumulated toxins. And it stimulates an enzyme system in the liver, which removes free radicals from the bloodstream. Coffee enemas were one of the great German discoveries in the 1920s. Gerson began using them in the '30s, and now many naturopathic disciplines use them as well."

"But why does the therapy take so long? Eighteen months seems an unconscionably long time to have to endure such deprivation."

"Well, Gerson believed that it takes approximately five to six weeks for each liver cell to divide and produce a healthier daughter cell. And for real liver health, perhaps fifteen new generations of increasingly healthier liver cells need to come into being."

"Not a cure for the fainthearted then," I observed. Rigorous and restricting, it seemed more than body or soul could bear: a sentence of eighteen months to two years, at the end of which one might or might not be cured. Yet, if one *were* cured…. After all, it had taken more than two years for my immune system to collapse.

"You must read Gerson's book," said Beata. "You can get it at the health food store on Baker Street. Skip the clinical bits—they can be heavy going. Just read the easier how-to sections. I'll give you Charlotte's phone number at the Gerson Institute in San Diego. Tell her you've spoken with me and ask when they can accommodate you."

Charlotte, I knew, was Dr. Gerson's daughter, who had been carrying on his work since his death in 1959.

"Oh, and you'll need a full-time helper when you return," added Beata, "to make the juices and prepare the organic meals. It's almost impossible to do this on your own, especially when you're having a flare-up."

"A flare-up?"

"A healing reaction—symptoms get worse, temporarily, as the healing process kicks in and toxins begin to move from the body fat into the bloodstream. That's when you'll need someone to keep the raw vegetable juices coming, because you'll be too ill to make them yourself."

I felt my courage begin to falter. I wasn't good at long-term suffering. Still, if I wanted to get well, I would have to bite the bullet, as Clive would say—or rather, bite the carrot.

"I'm glad you've decided to take the plunge," said Beata, as we walked to the door. "I'm sure you'll find it's the right step."

"I hope so," I replied, "because if it isn't…."

"And now that you'll be joining the club," she added, as we embraced, "don't you think we should be seeing a bit more of each other?"

The next day I went to Baker Street and bought Gerson's book, *A Cancer Therapy: Results of Fifty Cases*. The cover bore an impressive tribute:

> *I see in Dr. Max Gerson one of the most*
> *eminent geniuses in medical history.*
> —Albert Schweitzer

Gerson, I learned, had cured Schweitzer's wife of lung tuberculosis, after conventional treatments had failed. Later, he cured Schweitzer of advanced diabetes when the theologian was seventy-five years old.

Returning home with my purchase, I was aware of reaching a crossroad similar to the one Beata had faced three years earlier. At least I had the advantage of knowing someone for whom the therapy had worked. Still, whether it would work for me was far from certain.

I stretched out on the sofa with the book and a bag of potato chips, relishing the guilty pleasure I always felt when reading a book during the day—the legacy of a mother who, when she saw me with my nose in a book, would say "Shouldn't you be improving yourself, dear, instead of just wasting time?"

I began my delicious waste of time by opening the book at random: *"The soil is our external metabolism,"* I read. *"It is not really far removed from our bodies."* I read on:

> Metabolism and immune system are gradually damaged over a long period of time by inadequate nutrition: food grown on a depleted, artificially fertilized soil that does not contain the necessary minerals; food deficient in proteins and potassium, made toxic by chemicals, processed and refined until it contains no live, active nutrients without which health cannot be maintained.

I stopped. The processed and refined chip in my mouth tasted suddenly stale, its chemical crunch a bit less satisfying than before. I turned the bag over and read the ingredients on the back: "Dehydrated ... partially hydrogenated ... artificial color...." I set the bag aside and read on.

> The malnourished body is then made even more toxic by environmental pollution; impure air and water, chemicals at large everywhere. Eventually, the hidden starvation and the accumulation of toxins combine to cause a breakdown in the body's defense system, so that a tumor can develop.

Gerson wrote this in the 1940s, concerned even then with ecological issues that are still being contested today in certain halls of denial. Yet he was not even the first to advocate pure food and water as the key to lasting health. In 1809, a Richard Lambe, M.D., of London, published a treatise on the successful treatment of cancer by a diet of fruits, vegetables, and pure water. Like Gerson, Lambe eventually extended his diet to include the treatment of other diseases.

Long before our latter-day health gurus made nutrition fashionable (and profitable), Gerson in Germany, Norman Walker in the United States, and others were preaching similar diets for the prevention and cure of degenerative diseases—preaching, moreover, to a deaf and scoffing medical establishment. Not much has changed. Then, as now, one could always tell the pioneer by the arrows in his back.

As Sir Almroth Wright phrased it in his well-known dictum:

> Each new idea in medicine has to pass through three stages:
> First, when it is regarded as ridiculous;
> Second, when doctors say "It may be possible, but where is the proof?";
> And third, when it is finally dismissed by everyone as obvious.

In the transcript of a talk Gerson gave three years before his death, he explained the evolution of his therapy. It began, he said, with his early success with tuberculosis. That led to patients with terminal cancer seeking his help, which in turn brought him patients with an increasing number of hopeless conditions.

> "I was forced into that," he observed wryly. "On the one side, the knife of the AMA was at my throat and on my back I had only terminal cases. If I had not saved them, my clinic would have been a death house. I learned that in tuberculosis and in all other degenerative diseases, one must not treat the symptoms. The body—the whole body—has to be treated."

One must not treat the symptoms! The words leapt up at me from the page. Here was a doctor, driven from his country and scorned in mine, saying something so sensible, yet so radical, it seemed like a revelation. I read on avidly, marking each passage that spoke to my condition.

Gerson maintained that most disease is the manifestation of an improperly functioning immune system; that if the body's metabolism can be restored, it will heal itself. All well and good, I thought, but he developed his therapy in the 1930s before the chemicals of war began to spread their pollution throughout the world. How could carrot juice restore a shattered immune system? How could a vegan diet remove the herbicides that I, a long-time vegetarian, had been consuming for years?

On July 23, I reached Charlotte Gerson on the telephone. Her strong, faintly accented voice sounded reassuring. I told her about my mastectomy in '74, and asked if she thought the therapy could purge the pesticides from my body.

"It can," she said, "if you haven't had chemotherapy or too many drugs."

"No chemo, fortunately, but too many tranquilizers and antibiotics, I'm afraid. Do you think the therapy could cure my allergies as well?"

"Of course. The process is the same. As father stressed, the therapy is 'nonspecific.' But I cannot promise you a quick cure. You must be prepared to stay on the therapy for some time."

"Longer than the eighteen months required for cancer patients?"

"I don't know. We can only judge that when you're here. But there are no quick fixes for the toxic body. It is a slow, hard slog that tests one's endurance to the limit. You should plan to stay at the clinic for at least three weeks," she advised, "because the initial detoxification can produce strong flare-ups, which it would be better to experience under the doctor's supervision."

We fixed August 26 for the date of my arrival. That would give me a week to spend with my widowed father in Los Angeles, instead of the four-week pilgrimage I made each summer. We would need those few days together before I went into purdah.

There was so much to do before the 26th I wondered how I would get it all done in time. Yet, once I had committed to the therapy, each step fell effortlessly into place—from purchasing a juicer from the US to arranging for a friend to lay in the store of vegetables in advance—even to finding a helper, a Portuguese woman whose long-time employer had just died and who could start in September when I returned.

With my restrictive diet only weeks away, I embarked on a manic food binge—sanctioned, I kept telling myself, by social engagements that kept me exposed to temptation and smoke-filled rooms. This posed a dilemma: my lungs or my social life? At one dinner party, my "spiritually evolved" hosts held forth on the dangers of pollution while puffing smoke over their proudly prepared organic fare. Their self-delusion was only marginally worse than my own, which refused to connect the kind of food I was feeding my body with its mounting rebellion.

CHAPTER SIXTEEN

In August, I began to be affected by something in the new flat as well, especially at night. If the flight to Mexico was not to become an emergency, I would need to find a bolt-hole for my remaining nights in London, so I booked a room in a small hotel off the Brompton Road for the week until departure.

I had been in bed but a short time when I became aware of the presence of an allergen in the room. Wearily, I got up and performed a sniff test, but I was unable to pin down the source. Was it organotins—chemicals found in most hotel furnishings, mattresses, and bed linens, which are toxic even in small quantities? Or was it some other odorless chemical impossible to detect? Whatever it was, I knew I couldn't stay.

It was too late to find another hotel, and I couldn't return home, so I got dressed and drove aimlessly through the streets of Fulham, fighting discouragement and aching for sleep.

Around ten o'clock a light rain began to fall. Finding myself on Manresa Road, I pulled over to the curb, released the Honda's reclining seat for the first time, and attempted to doze. While the rain drummed monotonously down, scenes from a distant past rose, merged, and dissolved behind my eyelids—a past in which I took vigor for granted, and health was an eternal birthright.

I saw the woman shopper in the lingerie department at Harrods who told me her skin was so sensitive the only material she could tolerate against it was silk. I saw myself at the dowsing convention in Vermont, eating a piece of carrot cake when a caftan with beads glided past me, chiding sweetly, "Dead food!" And I saw the roadside spit in a Turkish village, where friends who had tasted the meat came down with food poisoning, which I had escaped.

Dawn crept through the rain-speckled windows. Stiff and unrefreshed, I returned the car's seat to its vertical position and drove home to shower and change. Then I rang Clive. I had already told him about the therapy—as much as he cared to know—so the news did not come as a surprise.

"I know now, Clive, that unless I can get these chemicals out of my body, I won't be able to live in this world, so this is my last hope."

"Well, my dear," he said, in a voice much warmer than usual, "I think you've made the right decision."

I suspected the warmth in his voice owed less to hope for my recovery than to relief at getting me off his back.

Later that morning, I returned to the hotel to let the manager know I would not be keeping the room. He didn't mind; the tourist season was underway.

"Oh, by the way," I said, "have you by any chance fumigated the beds recently?"

He looked alarmed, as though anticipating a bedbug complaint. "No, but we do that once a year. They were fumigated in January. Why?"

"Oh. Then perhaps that explains it."

"Explains what?"

"Well, you see … I'm chemically sensitive, and I may have been affected by the fumigant you used, whatever it was."

"But you couldn't have been," he laughed. "That was seven months ago!"

"Oh, yes … of course," I said, and let it go at that.

I found a room as a paying guest in the flat of a woman who lived across the square. Lying awake that night in a stranger's bed so near to my own, I tried not to think what would happen if I returned from Mexico even more sensitive than I was now, unable to live in my flat again—or anywhere else, for that matter—save, perhaps on a desert island. Yet I *had* to be in my home to do the therapy. I couldn't decamp each night with a 60-pound juicing machine, a Portuguese helper, and a bag of carrots.

Two days before departure, I rang Beata.

"Just as a precaution, Beata, in case the Portuguese lady lets me down, do you know someone here who could help with the juices for a week or two when I return?"

"There's a man here who gets people started on the therapy," she said, "but with so many cancer patients needing help, I'm sure you'll agree their need takes priority." Priority? Who but the most desperate sufferer would embark on such a Draconian regime? "You should start the coffee enemas immediately," she advised. "You'll need a quart of the coffee liquid, and be sure to lie on your right side. The reason for this is so the coffee will turn the corner of the colon from the descending to the transverse colon at the splenic flexure."

I wasn't sure I liked the sound of those descending and transverse tubes. I only hoped Max Gerson knew what he was about when he added this coffee lark to his therapy. Not that I was averse to the idea of enemas; having been spared them as a child, I had no hang-ups about them, so to speak, but neither did I know how to go about the procedure. When I asked Beata what to do, her mirth was so humiliating I felt too stupid to persist ("Surely you have the wit to figure it out for yourself; read Gerson's book!").

I flipped through his book, but he must have assumed that most people knew the drill. I bought an enema bag and prepared the brew, then wondered at what height the thing should be hung. The bathroom doorknob looked too low, and with no alternative hook of a suitable height, I suspended it from a four-foot standing lamp in the study. This caused such an inrush—and outrush—of liquid, the whole enterprise ended in disaster and stomach cramp.

Beata might have warned me! I thought crossly, as I tidied up the floor.

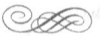

I flew to Los Angeles on August 17 with my usual headache, spurning the painkillers that would only have added to the chemicals I was hoping to shed. When I called the Gerson Institute to confirm my arrival on the 26th, the coordinator said:

"If you can be here by half past eight in the morning, Charlotte will drive you to the clinic herself, since it's one of her visiting days. By the way," he added, "will you have trouble negotiating the stairs?"

I explained that I didn't have cancer, I had pesticide poisoning, which manifested primarily as multiple allergies.

"Oh, allergies can take much longer to cure than cancer," he said. "Once your immune system has been repaired, you may have to remain on a modified version of the therapy for years."

Ah, well, I thought, so much for priorities.

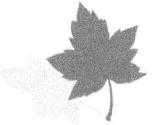

CHAPTER SEVENTEEN

I was standing outside the Gerson Institute when a car drove up and a tall, gray-haired woman stepped out.

"You must be Faye," she said, advancing with outstretched hand. "Hello, I'm Charlotte Gerson."

She was much as I had imagined her to be from her voice on the phone—the commanding presence, the calm authority, the quick mind, but with the added surprise of inquisitive blue eyes. I humped my suitcase, typewriter, and portable air purifier into the back seat of her car, and we set off for the Mexican border.

Charlotte asked after Beata, whose glowing health and warmest greetings I was delighted to convey.

"About your symptoms," she said. "I understand they manifest primarily as allergies?"

"Well, my main problem is pesticide poisoning," I said. "It seems to have made me hypersensitive to some peculiar things."

"Such as?"

I told her about my problem with crystals, earth energies, and the polluted stream, expecting the usual reaction, but I needn't have worried. Dowsing has a long and respected tradition in Germany, and Charlotte was as knowledgeable about the arcane as she was about cancer.

As our car crossed the border, I noticed a marked change in the landscape. The neatly groomed houses surrounded by greenery gave way to scenes of dust and disrepair. Clusters of Mexican *favelas* sprawled on a hillside, their makeshift materials festooned with lines of colorful washing—the garlands of poverty. Clapped-out American cars rattled along the pockmarked road, some with dented fenders and one with a bumper hanging half-off.

My interest in the scenery was only intermittent, however, for I was more interested in what Charlotte was saying. I had asked her why the clinic was in Mexico instead of California.

"It's in Mexico," she explained, "because it's against the law in California to treat cancer by any means other than surgery, radiation, or drugs, even though nutrition is safe and has no side effects."

"But why was such a law passed?" I asked. "In whose interest could it be?"

"The pharmaceutical companies, of course," she replied. "They have powerful lobbies in every state, and the American Medical Association is in their pocket. Its journal relies heavily on their advertising revenue, so the chemical companies got our lawmakers to rule that to treat cancer you can only slash, burn, or poison. But then you know this yourself, don't you?" she added, referring to the mastectomy I had mentioned on the telephone.

"But wasn't the purpose of the law to protect gullible people from quacks?"

"Of course there are quacks in every profession," she said. "But what about the patients who die *after* having surgery and radiation, or who suffer terrible side effects from chemo, and *still* die in the end? Ninety-five percent of the patients we see here are terminal cases. They come to us only *after* having been treated by orthodox doctors—who, by the way, have taken a fortune from them, yet nobody calls those doctors quacks."

I glanced at the handsome woman next to me, this latter-day St. Joan who was fighting the same battles her father had fought against an entrenched monopoly forty years earlier and lost. It was sobering to reflect that if Jesus returned tomorrow and fetched up in this land of the free, he could be arrested for practicing medicine without a license. Where were the civil liberties groups when the laws curtailing our freedom of medical choice were being enacted?

"Well, here we are," said Charlotte, swinging the car through a broad gate and into the forecourt of La Gloria Hospital. Compared to the arid landscape through which we had passed, La Gloria was an oasis, with well-kept greenery surrounding the buildings and a reassuring aspect of order.

We stopped in front of two long, low, single-story buildings, beyond which were a flight of steps that led to a larger two-story structure.

"That's the main building," said Charlotte. "This is the annex and the administrator's office."

She led me inside to register and receive an information folder. On the wall a large portrait of Dr. Gerson looked down on us, his expression sober, his keen blue eyes intelligent, observing. He had a look of stubbornness about him, but of kindliness as well.

"Come with me," said Charlotte. I followed her through the corridor of the annex to a room at the very end. "Will this be quiet enough for you?" she asked, opening the door to invite my inspection. I had asked Charlotte for a quiet room, since I hoped to do some work while I was there.

"It will be perfect," I said….

"You might like to know that this was Beata's room when she was here," said Charlotte, smiling. I laughed. Not only was I following in Beata's footsteps, like an aging Goldilocks I was sleeping in her bed as well.

"You'll find distilled water in the cooler outside the door," said Charlotte. "It's the only kind we use here."

She left me to unpack, and I surveyed my surroundings. They were those of any modest motel, save for the plastic-covered bench at the foot of the bed, which had an iron pole attached at one end with a double hook at the top for the enema bucket. A circular curtain, suspended from a track above the bench, could be drawn around it for privacy.

On a hot plate beside the bed, a carafe of coffee was being kept warm. How many caffeine addicts, I wondered, had broken the "no coffee by mouth" rule and secretly quaffed the odd cup?

Beata had warned me that the facilities at La Gloria were fairly primitive, but I didn't mind. What did concern me were the synthetic fabrics in the room: the PVC-covered bench, the polyester sheets and pillowcases—even a soft plastic cover on the toilet seat in the bathroom—and my nose began to recoil from the strong smell of disinfectant.

I began to unpack, removing my dowsing rod and color wheel, which I had brought to check the bed for any hostile energy lines. Happily, the room dowsed quiet. Just then, a small desk arrived, which Charlotte had kindly arranged for me to borrow. It took up most of the limited space in the room, but accommodated my electronic typewriter, diary, and writing materials.

I was hanging up my clothes when I heard a knock at the open door. I turned to see a short, gray-haired woman in a white coat standing in the doorway.

"Good morning," she said, "I am Dr. Melendez, the doctor assigned to your case."

Her round smiling face was a welcome change from some of the toffee-nosed doctors I had met in London. We reviewed my medical history together, and she had begun to do the preliminary blood tests when a girl appeared at the door with a glass of carrot and apple juice.

"Patients are put on the therapy as soon as they arrive," explained Dr. Melendez. Moments later, a plate of fruit and three thermoses arrived. "One thermos contains peppermint tea, one chamomile tea, and the third oat gruel," she said. "You should drink as much of these as you can and eat as much fruit as possible throughout the day."

I was savoring the taste of the organic carrot juice—so much sweeter than the commercial variety—when I noticed the fruit plate was tightly covered with Saran wrap, its plasticizers leaching into the organic produce. I pointed this out to Dr. Melendez and explained my concern. She looked surprised.

"I will have to tell them about that," she said. If she did, nothing was done about it while I was there.

By lunchtime, I had tasted the green leaf juice as well—a combination of vegetables chosen for their high potassium content: romaine lettuce, Swiss chard, green pepper, red cabbage, leafy beet tops (but not beets), and apple. I had also tried the carrot and raw liver juice, which tasted like soap. (This would be discontinued in '89, when it was no longer possible to find calves that hadn't been fed the hormones and steroids given to cows.)

Dr. Melendez left, and a pretty young nurse, Lulu, arrived to show me how to take an enema. Dimpled and smiling, she chattered away in Spanish, while explaining with hand gestures how high to hang the bucket, which I had finally figured out for myself.

Cheerful Lulu was followed by an older nurse who gave the daily injections of crude liver extract with vitamin B12. "You will be administering these injections yourself when you return home," she said. The scent of her perfume was so strong I could hardly breathe while she was in the room. How on earth was I going to detoxify in a place that was so indifferent to environmental hazards?

On entering the dining hall for lunch, I was struck by the air of cheerfulness in the room. If I hadn't known these were cancer patients, I would have taken them for a group of friendly tourists on holiday. None of the patients I met had "spurned the chance of a cure by choosing the alternative path first," to quote a radio doctor who spurned everything alternative. Each person at my table had undergone surgery, chemotherapy, and radiation, and still their cancers had returned. Only then did they come to Mexico as a last resort.

Some of the tales of medical mismanagement beggared belief. A young farmer from the Midwest, Randy, his stomach badly distended with leukemia, told his story.

"One doctor put me on Myloran® without discussing the side effects," he said. "He didn't even ask me to sign the required release form, which said that I understood the risks involved. After taking the damn pills for two days, I felt worse than I did from all the drugs I'd ever taken before— and that includes the hard stuff. I was puking and had a jackhammer headache that wouldn't go away, so I stopped taking it and flushed the rest down the toilet.

"But then I got curious and looked it up in the PDR (Physician's Desk Reference), and guess what I found: two columns devoted to Myloran's potential side effects, one of which was melanoma. And this," he snorted, "was being given to someone who had leukemia! Not only that, it had been listed as an experimental drug for forty years!"

Randy's story was so harrowing I didn't know whether to weep or rage. Had his oncologist been an alternative practitioner, he would have been hauled before a medical board and struck off for malpractice.

"And I'll bet you didn't know that no scientific double-blind studies have ever been done on chemotherapy drugs, either," he added.

"But why does your Food and Drug Administration *approve* such dangerous drugs?" asked Tina, a pediatrician from England who'd had a colostomy and now had cancer of the liver.

"Because they have a revolving door with the pharmaceutical companies," said Randy's brother, who was there as his caregiver. "Their officers land cushy jobs with the drug companies when they leave the government, so they spend our tax dollars trying to put alternative therapies out of business."

"I've often wondered," mused Tina, "if my original cancer could have been caused by an exposure to insecticides I had about five years before my diagnosis."

"Perhaps I can answer that," I said, venturing to join the discussion. "Five years seems about the time it takes for cancer to develop after a severe chemical exposure. The reason I know this," I added, eager to establish my right to be there, "is that I had breast cancer, and my immune system began to collapse from pesticide poisoning about five years before it was diagnosed."

A schoolteacher from Australia, Hal, spoke up, saying that he, too, had had a colostomy.

"I now have cancer of the rectum," he said. "When my doctor told me my condition was terminal, I decided to come here, although it's probably too late for me to expect a miracle."

"I'll show you a miracle," said Morris, an affable Canadian in his 70s and the senior member of our group. Standing up, he placed one foot on his chair and pulled his trouser leg up to the knee to display a slightly discolored shin. "I've had a gangrenous skin condition on both legs for thirty years," he boasted, "and it's almost gone since I started the therapy six months ago, see?" He added that his diabetes and prostate cancer were healing nicely, too. Morris, I learned, was the clinic's longest-staying resident—not because he needed to stay, but because he'd fallen in love with Mexico and gone native in a senior-citizen sort of way, studying Spanish and attending the local celebrations.

An American woman, Pearl, whose elderly husband was the patient, had been itching to speak. Thin and angular, with kohl-smudged eyes and frizzy bleached hair bunched over her forehead like a poodle's, she clinked and winked with silver jewelry, large rings on every finger.

"Harry's prostate cancer came back after chemo, too," said Pearl. "When he told his doctor he was going to come down here, the doc had a fit and tried to talk us out of it, but I told him what he could do with his chemo!"

With her raucous voice and quenchless energy, Pearl brought a liveliness to our table that was missing in her wizened spouse, whose emaciated arm she clung to with a quite unnecessary possessiveness.

And then there was Nora, whose husband, David, had pancreatic cancer, which had returned after chemo and now had metastasized to his bones. To this quiet, middle-aged couple from Montana I felt instantly attuned, so I was sorry to learn they were nearing the end of their stay.

The food at La Gloria was organic, vegetarian, and delicious, with a wide variety of dishes to choose from. Two items were served twice a day: the "Hippocrates" soup—a blend of vegetables chosen for their cleansing effect on the kidneys—and a baked potato. A bottle of flaxseed oil stood on each table, with a dish of peeled garlic cloves flanked by a press. Any therapy that *urged* you to eat garlic, I reckoned, couldn't be wrong.

No bread or dairy products were allowed for the first six weeks. ("The Gerson patient does not fill up on bread," read a stern fiat in the primer.) However, we were encouraged to eat and drink as much of the permitted foods as possible. My only complaint at the end of two weeks was that there was so much food I would have welcomed a day of fast.

Each patient received a sectioned pillbox containing the supplements we were to take in a certain order and at specific times during the day. These included niacin, thyroid, and pancreatin tablets, with Acidoll capsules (hydrochloric acid) to aid digestion. Liquid potassium compound was added to every serving of carrot juice—the juices were delivered hourly to our rooms—with a drop of Lugol's solution (iodine) added six times a day.

Plunged into a regime that ignored food rotation and flooded the system with the same vegetables and fruits day after day, I wondered how my body would respond to this radical change of direction. Halfway through lunch, my face, arms and bottom broke out in red, stinging splotches, like an angry heat rash.

"Don't worry," said Nora, who was sitting next to me, "It's the niacin flush. It goes away after twenty minutes or so."

"How soon do you think I'll have a flare-up?" I asked her.

"I can't really say," she replied, "it's different with each person, but I would think within a week."

Nora, who could see I needed looking after, reminded me after lunch that it was time for my first "coffee break," the Gerson euphemism for enema time.

"Be sure to hang the sign with the cup of coffee on the door," she said. "That way, if it's time for a juice, they'll know to leave the glass outside your room. They keep it covered to preserve the precious enzymes, because these deteriorate rapidly."

With so much to learn, I decided to make a list of the questions I needed to ask Charlotte when she stopped by later on her postprandial visit to the patients' rooms.

"Don't four coffee enemas a day destroy the lining of the colon?" I began, after switching on the tape recorder Beata had advised me to bring ("Your conversations with Charlotte will be important morale boosters when you return to England.")

"Not at all," Charlotte replied. "You see, to initiate healing, you have to detoxify the body, especially the liver-bile system. Caffeine dilates the bile ducts and stimulates the discharge of built-up toxins. And the fruit and freshly pressed raw vegetable juices stimulate the kidneys to detoxify the body. At the same time, because they're rich in minerals, enzymes, and vitamins, they start the process of returning these substances to the depleted organs."

"But wouldn't it be easier simply to take capsules with the requisite vits and mins?"

"No," said Charlotte. "You see, it's not the vitamin A in the carrots that is beneficial, as most people think; it's the *natural* beta-carotene that activates the immune response. If you have a severely toxic and damaged system, you can't absorb and utilize concentrated pills. In fact, they tend to irritate a terminal patient further and cause him to lose more of his own depleted reserves."

"By the way," I said, thinking longingly of potato chips, "why is salt forbidden on the diet?"

"Because sodium is an enzyme inhibitor," Charlotte explained. "In nature, all foods grow with the proportion of potassium to sodium that the body needs, sometimes as much as a thousand times more potassium than sodium. When foods are processed, they're cooked in such a way that the potassium is lost. So the average diet is heavily unbalanced, with far too much salt."

"Which contributes to high blood pressure?"

"High blood pressure returns to normal in five days on the therapy."

I showed Charlotte the antigen vaccines Jean advised me to keep taking.

"Is there a freezer where I could store these while I'm here?" I asked.

Charlotte eyed the vials warily. "You can take those if you want," she said, "but I don't think you'll need them when the therapy gets under way. We don't have a freezer here because all the food is fresh. The nurses have a refrigerator in their quarters with a small freezing compartment, which I'm sure they'd let you use. How many antigens do you have?"

"About fifty, ten in each vial."

Charlotte reached for a vial and read the ingredients on the label.

"Personally," she said, handing it back to me, "I don't feel good about injecting chemicals into the body, no matter how diluted they are."

"The antigens did help for a while," I said, "but then they seemed to stop working."

"Precisely. Because desensitizing vaccines are still just treating the symptoms and not the disease. They desensitize the body, but they don't rebuild its capacity to heal itself, nor do they detoxify. And, as my father said, 'Without detoxification, you cannot heal.' "

Persuaded by the logic of her argument, I decided to forgo the antigens while I was there.

I was in mid-enema the next morning, bare backside to the door, when I heard a knock, and before I could answer, a young man in a white coat entered.

"Good morning!" he said, in a cheery American voice. "My name's John. I'm an assistant here. I've brought you your supplements for the day."

He placed the box on the desk before turning to address me in a matey manner. "So, how're you doin'?"

"Um … fine," I said, stiff with embarrassment.

"Great! Well, see you tomorrow then," he said, and was gone.

Tomorrow, I vowed, that curtain will be drawn around the bench.

La Gloria could be an unsettling place for the intensely private person. Beata must have hated it.

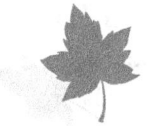

CHAPTER EIGHTEEN

"It looks as though Hal is having a setback," said Morris, noting Hal's absence at breakfast the next morning. Nora and David, too, were missing.

"I'm worried about him," said Tina. "He hasn't been doing at all well, and he's so alone here. I think we should look in on him, Morris, don't you?"

Tina, whose English reserve bordered on coolness, appeared to have a soft spot for Hal, perhaps because of their mutual colostomies or because they were both Brits. Turning to me, she said, "Won't you come with us?"

I wanted to decline, but was afraid of seeming standoffish, so I followed them into the annex where I discovered that Hal's room was two doors down from mine. We found him propped up in bed, looking like death, and surrounded by those emblems of the sickroom: damp towels on the floor, an open Bible on the nightstand, and next to it a glass of carrot juice, untouched.

Hal's face brightened when he saw us. "I've been running a fever since lunch yesterday," he said in a hoarse whisper. "Can't eat anything … the juices … can't get them down."

Tina and Morris chatted with Hal, their visit bringing him evident pleasure, while I stood by, feeling awkward and irrelevant, like the new girl at school invited to join an established clique.

After some minutes, Tina glanced at her watch. "Oh dear, Hal," she said, "it's time for my coffee break. I'm in the upper building, so I'll have to make tracks if I'm not to fall behind schedule."

"Me, too," said Morris. "We'll look in on you again, Hal, if we don't see you at breakfast tomorrow."

I moved to join them, but Hal said, "Oh please don't go—unless you must. It's so good to have company."

I wanted to leave, but he looked so ill and so lonely I didn't have the heart to refuse. Shifting his bathrobe from the chair to the table, I drew the chair up to his bed, hoping that Hal would do most of the talking.

"Tell me about yourself, Hal," I said. "I believe you were a teacher. What did you teach?"

"I taught chemistry," he said, and went on to tell me about his family, the onset of his cancer, and his fear the disease had spread too far to be reversed. At one point his voice faltered, he grimaced, and beads of sweat broke out on his brow. Without thinking, I reached over to feel his forehead. "Oh," he murmured, covering my hand with his, "that feels so good … a cool hand on my forehead."

I smiled. My hands were always cold; Reynaud's disease, the doctors said. Well, at least it could serve some useful purpose.

We sat in silence for a while, thinking our separate thoughts, neither one feeling the need to speak. I glanced at his open Bible noting the passages underlined in red and remembering how I did the same thing when I was a young and ardent Christian Scientist. Had someone told me then that I would be sitting in a cancer clinic one day feeling closer to God with the terminally ill than I had ever felt in church, I would not have believed them.

My mind was wandering thus, when I became aware of a strange queasiness in my stomach. Surely it was too soon to be having a flare-up. What, then, could be causing this strange malaise? I was wondering what to do when something an astrologer told me in London: "You must never enter the nursing profession," she warned. "You're too vulnerable, like an emotional sponge. You absorb other people's problems and can't help being affected by them—physically as well as emotionally."

At the time this struck me as hugely funny, for I was being affected by almost everything in the universe. Now, however, I wondered if my hand could be absorbing Hal's symptoms—the way it appeared to absorb the Dacron energy from the box of vials that day at the clinic.

Whatever the cause, I knew I couldn't stay.

"Hal," I said, after a suitable interval, "I'm afraid it's my coffee break time now, so I'll have to go. But if you would like me to stop by again on my way to dinner I will."

"Please do," he whispered—adding, feebly, "for another laying on of hands?"

The heat in my room was oppressive. I fell exhausted onto the bed. Only then did I think of my right foot, which had been swollen when I woke up that morning. I had forgotten about it in my preoccupation with Hal. Now, however, I noticed the edema had reached my ankle.

Dr. Melendez arrived a short time later. Seeing my prostrate form on the bed, she said, "You feel fatigued because of the potassium drops in the juices. Your body isn't accustomed to such a sudden correction of pH imbalance, a change from acidic to alkaline."

Then that could explain my queasiness, I thought, relieved.

"Could I skip a couple of juices today?" I pleaded. "I'm not sure I'll be able to keep them down."

"No," she said. "It is important to adhere to the therapy if you possibly can. One cannot skip the more difficult parts. Those who have tried to do this do not heal well." I drew her attention to my swollen foot and ankle. "You must have had an injury to that foot at some time," she observed, "because the swelling is a sign the healing reaction has begun. The allergic inflammation is vital to the healing process."

Injury to my foot? Then I remembered: my toe operation ... the swollen calf ... the forgotten suture.

Dr. Melendez left to continue her rounds, and I fell asleep. When I woke, I found I had slept through lunch and two juices, which were waiting, covered, outside my door, their enzymes almost certainly gone.

I recalled that Norman Frye, co-director of the institute, was giving a talk that afternoon, so I forced myself to get up. ("You will find the lectures wonderfully educational," Beata had said.)

Frye was speaking when I arrived, so I slipped into a seat at the back. A man in his 50s, with sandy hair and a neat moustache, Frye was talking about an eight-year-old patient, a Hungarian boy, Tamas, who had been cured of Ewing's sarcoma.

"This is a diffuse endothelial myeloma that forms tumors on long bones, for which the medical prognosis is very poor," Frye explained. "The boy was treated with chemotherapy prior to coming to Mexico, but the cancer spread from his pelvis into the soft tissues. He was pale and thin and had lost his hair when he came to us, but he was surprisingly well-disciplined and willing to eat the unsalted vegetarian food and drink the juices. He continued the regimen when he returned home and now, after two years, he's a strong and healthy lad of ten.

"What makes his recovery even more dramatic," Frye added, "is that he was one of seven children with Ewing's sarcoma who were being treated with chemotherapy in the same Hungarian hospital. Unfortunately, the six other boys died."

Later, I learned it was Beata who met the children's mothers while on a visit to Hungary and had urged them to try the therapy. Only Tamas's mother had decided to risk the nutritional path.

Since patients were encouraged to ask questions, I raised my hand and asked: "How does a child so young get cancer?"

For a moment Frye seemed discomposed. "Well," he said, "we won't go into that now."

His response surprised me. Why not go into it now? Surely we need to know why the incidence of cancer in children is rising. Did the mother smoke while pregnant? Did she do drugs? Was she exposed to chemicals?

Seventy years ago, cancer in children was almost unheard of. In 1962, Rachel Carson observed:

> A quarter-century ago, cancer in children was considered a medical rarity. *Today, more American school children die of cancer than from any other disease.* (Italics hers.)

My query went unanswered, for Frye had moved on and was now addressing the subject of flare-ups.

"These can occur at any time" he said, "within days or weeks of starting the therapy. They are the body's attempts to detoxify and heal itself, and the first flare-ups are usually the worst. Gradually, they'll become shorter and milder, until they disappear altogether. But the symptoms can be nasty at the beginning," he warned. "Old scars and wounds may turn red, arthritic joints may become inflamed and swollen, and headaches, weakness, and such may grow worse for a while. Old drug deposits, too—whether from aspirin or LSD—when being flushed from the body fat into the bloodstream, can produce a stronger effect than when they were being absorbed over a period of time.

"In sum," he concluded, "you are being asked to take charge of your own medical care, but you are being given nature's tools with which to do the job. Unfortunately, many are unable or unwilling to make the required changes in their lives. As difficult as the days ahead may be, I urge you not to panic when flare-ups occur, because they are signs the immune system is beginning to reactivate its defenses."

By the end of the lecture my nausea had gone, but I was still feeling tired, so I returned to my room and slept until dinnertime. On the way to the dining room, I looked in on Hal, who was no better, so I sat with him for a few minutes. How lonely he must be, I thought, so far from home, with no loved ones near. How I wished my hand could heal sickness, instead of absorb it.

My thoughts were running in this vein, when my inner voice whispered, He's not going to make it. It's too late; he needs hospice care. Yet hospice was for those who have accepted death; Hal was clinging to this last desperate chance for life. A great sadness came over me then, which I could not shake off for the rest of the evening.

At dinner I sat next to a woman who told me she was there as a caregiver for her friend, Marie, who had breast cancer.

"When the doctors found the cancer had spread," she said, "they removed some lymph nodes from under her arm, which caused severe lymphedema. I think the procedure is called an 'axillary node dissection.' When we arrived here ten days ago, Marie's arm was so swollen it stuck out at a right angle to her body. She couldn't dress herself or comb her hair or do anything, which is why we've been having our meals brought to the room. The swelling has almost gone now, and some dark stuff has started to come out around the nipple on her breast. The doctor says it's the dead cancer cells exiting through her pores."

This was so hard to believe I asked if I could meet Marie after dinner.

She was sitting up in bed reading when we arrived. A good-natured woman in her fifties, she responded willingly to my questions, showing me how swollen her arm had been before by lifting it straight out to the side, as though directing traffic.

"See?" she said, letting her arm fall. "Now the swelling is gone and I can even comb my hair again. And look at this," she added, drawing the top of her robe to one side to reveal her breast and the dark crusts that had formed around the nipple. "The dead cancer cells are coming out through my skin."

Had I not seen this myself, I doubt I would have believed it. Yet I had been reading a book by an earlier Gerson patient, Jaquie Davison, who, like Beata, had been cured of melanoma. She, too, described the dead cancer cells coming out through her skin, only hers had exited through the soles of her feet. How I wished I had known about the therapy when I had breast cancer. In the few days I had been at the clinic the edema in my foot had subsided, my hair had regained some of its curl, and if there were noxious energy lines at La Gloria, I wasn't aware of them.

Returning to my room I found two small paper cups sitting on the desk. One held brown sugar, the other castor oil. I knew they were for the castor oil enema in the morning, but I wasn't sure when or how to take them, so I rang the nurse's office for advice. A woman answered in Spanish.

"Habla Ingles?" I asked, in my high-school Spanish.

"Si, si," said the voice and hung up.

Assuming someone would ring back, I waited. And waited. When forty minutes had passed, I gave up and went to bed. Thank God it wasn't an emergency, I thought. This *mañana* way of life takes some getting used to.

When John arrived at six the next morning (my coffee break postponed until after his departure), I asked, "What am I supposed to do with the castor oil?"

"You should have taken it at five this morning, along with the coffee in the thermos. Didn't they bring you any?"

"No."

"I'll have them send you some. The cup contains two tablespoons of castor oil. If you knock it back with the coffee, you won't taste a thing. Your regular enema is taken an hour later. Four hours after that, you do the castor oil enema. That's what the extra bucket is for."

I had no problem downing the castor oil, but the enema five hours later was a misery to administer. For the viscous liquid to slide down the hose, it had to be mixed with castile soap and be constantly stirred with a wooden spoon until the bucket was drained. The result—not to put too fine a point on it—felt like giving birth to an elephant. Trust a Teuton, I thought, albeit a Jewish one, to devise a cure that attacks the colon.

By contrast, I quite enjoyed the coffee enemas, for apart from the sense of well-being they provided, they offered twenty minutes of quiet reading time. Much of my education in nutrition, the environment, and the spiritual subjects I was exploring took place while I was lying on a bench in Mexico with my nose stuck in a book and a hose stuck up my backside.

Why, I wondered, have enemas received such a bad press? In an age when no aspect of sex is taboo nor any orifice a mystery; when pornography is available at the click of a mouse and we've even had a president who taught sixth graders the meaning of oral sex, it does seem a bit prissy to go all squeamish at the thought of cleansing the colon.

Charlotte was waiting for me when I returned to my room after lunch. I switched on the tape recorder and, thinking of Hal, asked her if she knew what the therapy's failure rate was.

"Well, you must realize," she said, "that almost all the patients we see here have metastasized cancers no longer treatable by orthodox methods, so of course there are failures. We have a high dropout rate as well. Not everyone has the self-discipline to stick with the therapy when the going gets rough. Some patients drop out after a few months because they can't cope with the flare-ups."

They had my sympathy, but I would not be one of them. When I committed to the regime, I promised myself that if it failed the fault would not be mine.

"But to answer your question," Charlotte continued, "As far as we can tell, we have a 20 to 30 percent success rate." (This was in 1985; the rate has grown since then as the therapy has expanded into other countries.)

I put to Charlotte the same question I had put to Norman Frye the day before.

"Charlotte, why do you think children are getting cancer at a younger and younger age? After all, they haven't lived long enough to have acquired a large toxic burden."

"One of the main problems is pesticides," she said, "but there are other reasons too. Fluoride in the water is one, but also immunization at six weeks, when they give the shot with diphtheria, pertussis, and tetanus. The dangers of the DPT shot have been thoroughly documented in a number of studies—all ignored by the immunization lobbies, of course." I thought of two couples I knew whose sons, normal at birth, had been brain-damaged after vaccination. One boy was now autistic, while the other was intellectually disabled and in a wheelchair.

Both had older sisters who were unaffected by the same vaccines, which made me wonder if the male immune system was weaker at birth than the female? I could not agree with Charlotte, however, that all immunizations were bad—after all, the Salk vaccine had virtually eradicated polio. Still, I was not prepared to challenge her on the subject, so I said, "I had no idea immunization was unsafe."

"You cannot believe how dangerous it is," said Charlotte. "The earlier it is done the worse, because the immune system is not developed yet in children. We saw a case like that some time ago. A young mother came as a companion to her father, who had cancer. Because she was nursing, she brought her baby along. But the baby, who was three months old, arrived in a state of respiratory distress.

"The mother told us that her pediatrician had recommended the shot at six weeks: 'Your baby's doing so well we can start the DPT shot.' Shortly afterward, the child had trouble breathing, and if you can't breathe, you can't nurse. So the mother—worried, but not suspecting the connection—went back to the doctor, who gave the child some drugs. And it got worse. So what do you do if drugs make a child worse? You give it *more* drugs, right?" she said acidly. "That's what the doctor did and *still* the child cried at night and couldn't sleep or nurse. This was the state she was in when they arrived here.

"Now, we didn't touch the child," said Charlotte. "We *never* treat a baby. But since this mother was nursing, we treated her. We put her on a lot of vitamin C and carrot juice, with potassium and enemas, and in three days the baby was fine."

"That's the most powerful argument I've heard for breast feeding and pure nutrition."

"Well, the therapy is not just a cure for cancer or for this or that disease," Charlotte reminded me. "By restoring and strengthening the *whole* immune system, it restores the body's ability to heal itself."

That may be true with cancer, I thought, but could it also purge the system of toxic chemicals?

"Ah, well," said Charlotte, rising, "I have more patients to see, so I'd better be on my way."

I switched off the tape recorder and rose. At the door she paused, turned, and with an air of infinite sadness, said, "What a world we live in, eh?" And then she was gone, her swift, determined footsteps echoing down the hall.

For a while I sat thinking about her: her courage, her selfless dedication, and the vast amount of knowledge she had acquired during the years she spent working at her father's side. I thought of her struggle to keep his therapy alive, and the encouragement she gave to every patient in the clinic, week after week, year after year.

And I decided that in my pantheon of saints, Charlotte Gerson stood very near the top.

CHAPTER NINETEEN

I had been reading Jaquie Davison's account of her healing of melanoma before there was a clinic to go to, when she had only Gerson's book to guide her. What kept me plodding through her religious effusions were the signs—of which she seemed unaware—of her exposures to chemicals. Although it was still early days, I was finding the regime less onerous than I had expected, but then I seemed to require a tight framework in order to achieve anything at all. Perhaps the diet was harder to follow for people with stronger addictions to relinquish, such as alcohol, tobacco, or drugs. My cravings were the childish ones for sweets and carbohydrates, but no less tenacious for that.

The road to health, alas, is paved with renunciation.

When Charlotte came for her visit on the twenty-ninth, I told her about my swollen foot and the suture left in one toe.

"That reminds me of a patient whose nose began to swell at the start of the therapy," she said. "Shortly thereafter, a suture appeared in one nostril. When I asked if she'd had a nose operation, it turned out she'd had a rhinoplasty thirty years earlier. She recalled that, two weeks after the operation, a small piece of suture stuck out from inside her nostril. Instead of pulling it out she had cut it off, and since it hadn't bothered her, she'd forgotten about it. Because the therapy helps the body expel any hostile substance, the tissue surrounding the remaining suture became inflamed and it made its way out of her body quite naturally.

"By the way," she added, "how many operations have you had—I mean with anesthetics and antibiotics?" When I told her five in one year, her hands flew to her face in mock horror. "Thank God they didn't give you chemo when you had cancer," she said, "because it destroys what is left of the immune system and makes it much harder for the therapy to work."

"That reminds me of a question I meant to ask you Charlotte, though I think I know the answer. Why are patients advised to take care of any dental work before they start the therapy?"

"Because the detoxifying body is too sensitive to tolerate anesthetic," she said.

I described my near-death experience in the dental chair, adding, "I understand the ECU has since been closed and Dr. Rae now has a sauna program instead."

"Well, saunas can sweat out some of the toxins," she said, "but not all poisons can be eliminated through the skin."

"I wonder why I felt so well after the four-day fast, only to have my symptoms return when I started eating single-food meals?"

"That's because your body was still full of poisons. Fasting gives temporary relief to an overloaded system, but it should not be applied in chronic disease because deficiencies are always present. My father opposed fasting as a detoxification procedure, since it doesn't restore the urgently needed minerals and vitamins to the organs. He didn't like spring water either—not only because much of it contains salt, but because the consistent purity of the spring can't be guaranteed. There is no way to protect a spring from pollution."

On this subject Gerson was even wiser than he knew. At the 1984 convention of the American Dowsers Society in Vermont, a professional water diviner told us he was having to go much deeper than before to find potable water, because the underground aquifers are being contaminated by agricultural chemicals. More worrying than the pollution of our food is the contamination of the world's water resources, because without pure water life on earth cannot be sustained.

As long ago as 1939, the French aviator Antoine de St. Exupéry wrote in *Terre des Hommes—(Man's Earth)*:

> The human body cannot go three days without water. I should never have believed that man was so truly the prisoner of the springs and freshets.... We believe that man is free. We never see the cord that binds him to wells and fountains, that umbilical cord by which he is tied to the womb of the world. Let man take but one step too many ... and the cord snaps.

That cord has been tightening for many years now, but only recently have we begun to realize how soon it could snap.

I asked Charlotte if she was familiar with the hospice movement in England that was doing such wonderful work for the terminally ill. At the word "hospice," she stiffened slightly and her manner changed.

"Yes, I'm familiar with the hospice movement," she said, "but that doesn't interest me." Seeing my surprise at her indifference, she added, "You know Elisabeth Kübler-Ross?"

"Of course." Kübler-Ross was legendary even in the '70s for her work in helping the dying come to terms with death. It was at one of her lectures in London that I learned about the hospice movement, which was pioneered in England by Dame Cicely Saunders.

"Now, Kübler-Ross is a wonderful woman," said Charlotte, "a *caring* woman, who is breaking down the taboos about death." She paused. "But I would not let her set *foot* in this place!"

Shocked by her vehemence, I said, "I don't understand, Charlotte, why wouldn't you?"

"Because I'm not interested in helping people to *die!*" she said, spitting out the word as though it were an obscenity. "We're only interested here in helping people to *live!*"

Her voice was so triumphant, so life-affirming, that I wanted to stand up and cheer. If Charlotte Gerson was a chip off the old block, what a sequoia the block must have been!

Frye's lecture that afternoon focused on Max Gerson's life, which had been one of high achievement plagued by tragic misfortune. Beata describes it so engagingly in her book that, with her permission, I am quoting part of it here:

> From my sketchy sources he came across as a strong, gentle, quiet man, absorbed in his work, absent-minded enough to wreck four bicycles in minor accidents and to fall down a coal chute. Above all he was modest, unpretentious and tenacious. Without exceptional staying power he might have packed up medicine altogether or suffered a breakdown in his prime, for his whole life was punctuated by tragic reverses and disappointments. It was as if Fate had offered him marvelous opportunities with one hand, only to snatch them back with the other just before fruition. Yet even with such a cruel stop-go pattern, Dr. Gerson had achieved unique results; what might he have done on a smoother track?
>
> Two episodes of his career stood out as particularly bitter milestones. In 1932, when he was fifty-one, he was granted full facilities at a Berlin hospital to prove that his dietary treatment could cure even hopeless cases of tuberculosis. After long and painstaking efforts he was due to demonstrate his results before the Berlin Medical Association, in a presentation that he knew would make his therapy widely accepted and open the door to further pioneering work. But five weeks before the scheduled demonstration Hitler came to power, and Dr. Gerson left Germany with his wife and three daughters. (Many of his relations who refused to follow his example perished in Nazi concentration camps.)
>
> Another dazzling opportunity came—and went—in 1946 when Dr. Gerson, by then resettled and working in New York, was allowed to present five of his recovered cancer patients to a U.S. Congressional committee, the first physician to be able to do so. What was at stake was a Senate bill that, if passed, would have provided funds for research into his therapy.

The presentation was an unqualified success, but the lobby supporting conventional cancer therapies defeated the bill by four votes. And that was that. The solitary immigrant doctor with his German-flavored English and remarkable results was once more left out in the cold, partly ignored, partly persecuted by various medical organizations, including the American Cancer Society, which listed his therapy under the heading of 'Frauds and Fables.' But he went on working, alone, amid increasing difficulties, and died at the age of seventy-eight, in 1959. As the final irony of his strange fate, the New York Academy of Science invited Dr. Gerson to become a member— two months after his death.

Only once did his life pattern seem to have worked in reverse when, instead of reducing a great chance to ashes, it turned a severe handicap into a tool of discovery. As a young man Dr. Gerson suffered from long, incapacitating bouts of migraine which his medical colleagues could not cure. So he began to experiment with various diets and soon found that a saltless regime of raw or freshly cooked vegetables and fruits, especially apples, banished his migraines. He recommended the same diet to his migraine-stricken patients, with excellent results. Soon one of those patients reported that his severe attacks of migraine had ceased—and his Lupus vulgaris (skin tuberculosis) was also healing. Since Lupus was considered incurable, Dr. Gerson could hardly believe the man's claim—or the evidence of his own eyes. But there could be no doubt. The Lupus lesions were healing. And he was forced to conclude that the diet was not so much healing a specific illness as restoring the body's own ability to heal itself—of migraine, Lupus, TB, or whatever was wrong with it. That was how his revolutionary work began, leading, in due course, to his startling success with terminal cancer cases.

When Gerson immigrated to America in 1936, he was fifty-five years old and spoke little English. To learn the language he went to school with first- and second-grade children, so he could pass the New York State board examination. He obtained his medical license in January 1938.

After Gerson's presentation before Congress was defeated, the *Journal of the American Medical Association* (*JAMA*) reported, "Fortunately for the American people, this presentation received little, if any, newspaper publicity." In January 1949, the same journal stated, "There is no scientific evidence whatsoever to indicate that modifications in the dietary intake of food or other nutritional essentials are of any specific value in the control of cancer." Thirty years later, the AMA was still claiming, "There is no proof that diet is related to disease."

Efforts to destroy Gerson did not stop at his therapy. Twice, he became violently ill after being served coffee by a group of people he was led to believe were supporting him. Laboratory tests showed arsenic in a 24-hour sample of his urine. Some of his best case histories disappeared mysteriously from his files, and in 1956, someone stole his almost-completed book manuscript.

Gerson was seventy-five years old and faced with rewriting his entire life's work. *A Cancer Therapy: Results of Fifty Cases* was published in 1958. In the fall of that year, he realized that, at seventy-seven, and in failing health, he would never finish his next book, which would present 100 more recovered cancer cases. He died of pneumonia in March 1959. Even then, the medical establishment claimed he had died of cancer, although his death certificate confirmed the cause.

What eminence might Gerson have achieved had he not been forced to flee his native land? How many life-saving cures were lost in the gas ovens of the Nazi extermination camps? Like so many pioneers, Gerson was an eccentric genius—unable or unwilling to conform to the prevailing norm. Too single-minded to care about image and too honest to cultivate charm, such visionaries can be prickly challengers of the status quo. Scorned by their peers and denied funding, after their deaths their work is appropriated—without credit—and claimed as "new" by the same sort of people who, when they were alive, were calling them quacks.

Not much has changed since Gerson's day. Medical McCarthyism still flourishes in America. The same obstacles Gerson faced in 1946 confront the heretical visionary today. Money and power protect the huge profits of the cancer industry—a cartel that continues to claim "There is no cure, but one is on the way."

Frye's lecture that day ended with a description of the latest craze of the '80s: fire-walking.

"It encourages people to run barefoot over burning coals as a way of conquering their fear," he explained. "Once you've done that—conquered a different kind of fear—you have more courage with which to face your cancer."

Well, perhaps. But cancer didn't scare me in 1974. Compared to the torment of telluric energies, skipping barefoot over hot coals was a game for masochistic morons.

"I will show you fear in a handful of dust," wrote T. S. Eliot. In the chemical spray from a crop duster's plane; in the toxic particulates that waft through the air; and in the terrible beauty of the mushroom cloud that one day may extinguish us all.

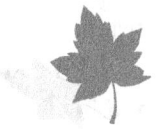

CHAPTER TWENTY

Two newcomers appeared at our table for dinner that evening, a quiet young man who suffered from asthma and his guitar-playing companion, a Texas evangelist in his thirties.

"Hi, there!" said the latter, rising mid-meal to address the room. "My name's Jimmy Jackson—*Pastor* Jimmy Jackson—and this here's my friend Roy, who's the patient. I understand it's someone's birthday today. Could you raise your hand, whoever you are? Oh, it's you over there. Well, c'mon, everyone, let's all sing 'Happy Birthday' to the birthday girl."

He seemed an odd companion for his reticent friend, who said hardly a word throughout dinner. With the pastor's guitar, his soft baby face, and brown hair combed in an upstanding quiff, he seemed more Elvis than evangelical.

"If I can be of help to any of you while I'm here," he added in his Texas twang, "you just let me know. Oh, and I'll be having a sing-along in the lounge after dinner for those of you who'd like to join me."

"Let's go to my room now, Nora, shall we?" I said. My typewriter had developed a glitch that afternoon, and being electronically challenged I had issued a distress call at dinner. To my surprise, Nora had said she was quite good at fixing things and offered to have a look at it. David, who was quieter than usual that evening, chose to return to their room.

It took Nora only a short time to detect the portable's problem and put it to rights. That done, we sat on the bed and had a quiet talk together.

"I'm so worried about David," she said. "He's not doing at all well. I think his cancer is too advanced now for anything to help. If only we had known about this option before he was given so much chemo." She paused, gazed into the middle distance, and said, "We've been married thirty-six years. It won't be easy ... letting him go."

I reached for her hand, wondering why shared sorrow brings us so much closer than shared joy. At such moments it was hard not to rail at the injustice of fate and the remoteness of God. But then, while Nora was speaking of her long, happy marriage and the future she dreaded without her husband, a curious illness stole over me and my thoughts grew muddled.

Noting my confusion, she asked, "Are you all right?"

"I think so—that is, I don't know. I'm feeling a bit odd."

"Perhaps you should lie down. Would you like me to call a nurse?"

"No, no, it will pass. Anyway, Nora, David needs you and you should be with him. He seemed to be having a hard time at dinner. But thank you again—for everything."

When she had gone I stretched out on the bed and tried to analyze my malaise. Was I having a flare-up? If so, it wasn't a very big one. I just felt ill and unconfident and alone.

My confusion cleared after a coffee break, during which I read more of Jaquie Davison's book. Reflecting on the strong family support she had while doing the therapy at home—a sympathetic husband and a daughter who took a year off school to make the juices for her mother—I realized why the regime, as it now stands, might not be widely used. In order for it to succeed, three things are essential:

1. Sufficient funds to pay for the juicer, supplements, and food.
2. Someone to make the juices and organic meals—a full-time, labor-intensive job.
3. Family support—or, failing that, the courage to go it alone.

It does not diminish Davison's achievement to say that without her strong support system at home, her outcome might have been quite different.

On August 30, the niacin flush made my bottom go all crimson, like the bum of those exotic monkeys in zoos who display themselves to snickering children. I still didn't know if I'd had a proper flare-up, apart from exhaustion on castor oil days.

"Don't you feel lonely down there in the annex?" Nora asked me at lunch. "You're missing a lot, you know, not being in the upper building. Why don't you take our room when we leave the day after tomorrow? It's larger than yours and much nicer. Then, too," she added, "you'd be closer to the nurses in case of an emergency." Seeing the wry look this comment elicited, she added, "Well, suppose you had an emergency down there at night all by yourself?"

"Oh, Nora, what could a nurse do for me, even if she spoke English? They only know cancer here, not chemicals."

"But I don't like to think of you being so alone."

Just then, Jimmy Jackson rose to make an announcement.

"Good afternoon, all. I'll be having a musical get-together after lunch, if any of you'd care to join me."

"Oh, very well, Nora," I said, "let's go have a look at your room. By the way," I added, as we were climbing the stairs, "I hope your room isn't near his."

"Oh, no, they're four doors away. Anyway, I was told he's been asked not to play his guitar in the evening, because the patients need rest and quiet."

"Well, that's a mercy," I said. Then, afraid of sounding judgmental, I added, "He's not a bad chap, it's just that I spent a month with a Baptist woman in Texas, and a little fundamentalism goes a long way."

The upper building was indeed more spacious, and its broad corridor was lined with chairs that invited communal visiting. On reaching their room, I was brought up short by the sign on the door: GOD IS LOVE.

"It was left there by a previous occupant," Nora explained. "You can remove it, if you want."

"I wouldn't dream of removing it," I said. "I used to see those words on the wall behind the lectern each Sunday in church. They make me feel right at home."

Not only was their room larger than my cubicle in the annex, it had its own water cooler as well. Much as I would miss Nora when she was gone, at least her vibrations would be around me.

The postprandial lecture that day was given by a German-born woman, Hildegard, who Charlotte described as "one of the sickest patients we've ever had." She visited the clinic once a week to inspire patients and instruct them on how to reorganize their kitchens when they returned home.

Hildegard told us her cancer began in 1977 with a tumor in her thymus the size of a grapefruit.

"When the doctors opened me up to remove it, they found that the tumor had invaded not only my thymus but my chest cavity as well. It had attached itself to my heart, aorta, trachea, and sternum. Since my condition was inoperable, they took a biopsy, closed me up, and gave me radiation—5,000 rads of cobalt to the thymus alone.

"After three weeks of this, I became violently ill, and I had severe burns on my esophagus and difficulty swallowing. The radiation caused my right lung to collapse and I developed pericarditis. My heart sac was full of pus, I had edema in my legs and throughout my body, and a liver scan showed spots of cancer."

When Hildegard came to the clinic, the doctor told her that not even the Gerson Therapy could help her and advised her to go home. But she said, "No, I've come here to get well, and I'm going to stay."

When she began the therapy in February 1979, she had hair loss, an enlarged liver, an immovable shoulder, a collapsed lung, and fluid in her lower lung and heart. Now, six and one-half years later, and in her fifties, Hildegard was the picture of health.

"I teach, work, and walk five miles or more every day. I do all my own housework and am about to go on a sailing trip with my son. If *I* could make it," she told us confidently, "so can you."

Yes, I thought, but only if we have your grit and determination.

On the first of September, I woke with strange new pains in different parts of my body. I had gone off food the day before and had skipped the last coffee break. I was tempted to cheat on the juices, too, but conscience kicked in and I forced them down.

After a sad goodbye to Nora and David in the morning, I began to pack for the move to their room. Since I couldn't carry my suitcase, typewriter and air purifier up the stairs alone, I rang the office to ask if there was someone who could give me a hand. "Si, si," said a woman, a "muchacho" would come right away.

While waiting for him to arrive, I went to see Randy, whose room was one door down from mine. He hadn't appeared at meals for two days, and we were concerned about him. I knocked gently and a young woman opened the door.

"Hello," she said. "I'm Randy's wife. My brother-in-law needed a break, so I came to take over. I'd invite you in, but he's not up to seeing anyone, I'm afraid. He's been in constant pain, lying on his stomach for the past two days, because one buttock is terribly swollen. He's been coughing up blood and his bed linens can't be changed because he's too ill to be moved."

Seeing my eyes slide down to the small knife in her hand, she blushed. "Oh, this," she said. "I've been cutting grapes into a bowl and putting them on the inflamed parts of his body as a poultice. Well," she added, "when you're desperate, you'll try anything, won't you."

Yes, I thought, as I walked back to my room, desperation has brought all of us here, some to find healing, while for others—often, it seemed, the most worthy—the journey had begun too late.

When an hour had passed with no sign of a muchacho, I went to the kitchen to see if someone there could help me. Eventually, a man whose muchacho days were long past came to take my suitcase and typewriter up the stairs, while I followed with my air purifier. He said he would bring the desk up later, but I never saw him again.

Moving day, Mexican style, was pretty much a do-it-yourself affair.

On September 2, Dr. Melendez brought me the results of my standard blood test. It was normal, except for low thyroid and a weak immune system.

"We'll have to do another blood test to see if your lymphocytes have gone up," she said. "These are the white cells that fight infection and disease. They should be between 20 and 40, but yours are below 10. So you'll have to remain on the full therapy."

"Precisely what I intended to do," I said.

The move to the main building proved to be a mixed blessing, the gain in space offset by the thinness of the walls, through which I could hear every movement in my neighbor's room, every footstep in the corridor, and every knock on someone else's door.

Meanwhile, the pastor's presence was beginning to cloy. Chatty and exuberant, unburdened by doubt or humility, he played his guitar, sang hymns, and offered his spiritual counsel to one and to all. Some of us were giving him a wide berth.

Returning to my room after the lecture that day, I caught sight of J.J. on the first floor, surrounded by the girls from the kitchen, singing a song whose words appeared to consist solely of *Vaya con Dios,* ad infinitum.

Two nights later, the sound of voices and laughter in the next room kept me awake after nine. I was wondering what to do, when the twang of a guitar brought me bolt upright in bed. *"Oh, no, God,"* I cried, *"you couldn't do this to me! Who can he be visiting at this hour? It's nearly ten!"* I reached for my earplugs and buried my head in the pillow, muttering darkly, *"Who will free me from this turbulent pastor?"* Someone Up There must have heard me, for a few minutes later, J.J. packed it in.

I was drifting off when a trolley came clattering down the corridor and stopped outside my window. Two maintenance men had chosen this hour to replace a light bulb in the ceiling—a task that required much animated discussion and scraping of the ladder on the tiled floor.

Yielding to fate, I shoved the earplugs in further, wrapped the pillow around my ears, and wished fervently that I had never left the annex.

CHAPTER TWENTY-ONE

I was heading for breakfast the next morning when I noticed the sign hanging on my neighbor's doorknob—the room J.J. had been visiting the night before: It pictured a set of headphones encircling the words, TUNED IN TO GOD! When I returned later the sign had been reversed; it now said, LISTEN! THERE'S GOOD NEWS IN JESUS!

The clinic was athrob with religious zeal.

Charlotte's postprandial talk that afternoon began by addressing the subject of stress.

"Stress does not cause disease," she said, flatly. "If it did, we would all be sick. It *can* be a precipitating factor if the body is already not functioning well and is deficient and toxic. Then, the addition of stress can be the straw that breaks the camel's back. But in a normal, healthy body, stress alone does not cause disease."

Returning to the subject of nutrition, she explained, "Chronic disease has two basic factors: deficiency and toxicity. Deficiency comes from our food, which is altered, processed, manufactured, canned, frozen, and so on. The vital live substances are gone. Toxins are enzyme inhibitors; so is sodium. Doctors in medical school aren't given courses in biochemistry, even though biochemistry is how the healing occurs. If correct nutrition can cure terminal cancers, imagine how few cancers there would be if we followed a healthy lifestyle from the start. Most of us are walking about in a state of half-health, believing ourselves to be well if we are not yet actually sick.

"And here I would like to say a word about soy. Soy is not a healthy food. It is a toxic by-product of the vegetable oil industry. Before soybeans reach your table, hexane or other solvents have been applied to help separate the oil from the beans, which leaves trace amounts of these toxins in the commercial product. Commercial soybeans block the absorption of any and all nutrients you take in. They also cause cancer of the thyroid. All soybean products contain trace amounts of carcinogenic solvents. They also contain much fat, which stimulates tumor growth."

Charlotte's lecture ended with a humorous story about a patient who had been on the therapy since her child was born.

"The patient's daughter was still young when she went to a friend's house for her first sleepover. On returning home the next morning, the little girl said, 'You know, Mommy, they do the strangest thing with coffee at her house—they *drink* it!'"

Returning to my room after the lecture, I was about to open the door when a voice said, "Hi there. I've got a surprise for you!" I turned to see Jimmy Jackson approaching. "You've got new neighbors," he beamed, withdrawing a key and inserting it in the door with the Jesus sign.

"You mean … this is *your* room?" I stammered.

"That's right."

Dear Jesus, this is not good news. Nora promised me! Forcing a smile, and with as much grace as I could muster, I said, "Well, I hope you won't be playing the guitar at night, Jimmy, because I turn in early and I'm a light sleeper."

"No problem," he said cheerfully. "If there's anything I can do for you, just let me know." He flashed a winning, if wasted, smile, and we entered our adjoining rooms.

True to his word, Jimmy did not play the guitar at night. He played it the next day. And sang. With his door open: "Drop Kick Me, Jesus, through the Goalposts of Life!"

My neighbor's occasional guitar riffs didn't bother me when I was writing in my diary or getting dressed, but if I was trying to read or work or *think*, they turned my brain into porridge. I could ignore the voices and laughter—even the odd resonant belch—but music was such a visceral part of my being I couldn't tune it out—especially the sort of "music" I would have gone some distance to avoid.

One morning, when those lachrymose twangs were making the effort to work like a slow tread through treacle, my tolerance threshold collapsed.

Marching into the corridor, I knocked on J.J.'s open door and walked in. He was reclining on the bed in a red dressing gown with his guitar. Roy sat sprawled in the armchair, doing nothing in particular.

"Jimmy," I began, "I know I'm not as ill as most of the patients here, but I *am* desperately in need of peace and quiet. If you must play the guitar, would you mind playing it somewhere else or moving to another room? I think there's an empty one at the end of the corridor."

He placed his guitar on the floor, propped himself up on his forearm and fixed me with a level gaze.

"I know there's an empty room at the end of the corridor," he said, "'cause that was our room before we moved here. But *you* can move, if you like," he added, a shade ungraciously, I thought.

"With the greatest respect, Jimmy, I'm a patient here and you're not. I'm simply asking you to show some consideration. By the way, may I ask *why* you changed your room?"

"We had to move 'cause there was no water in the shower and we got tired of waiting three days for it to get fixed."

"I see." There was no answer to that, so—after obtaining his promise of restraint, I returned to my room, cursing Mexican plumbing, cursing the *mañana* culture, and cursing my infernally low noise threshold.

Frye's lecture that afternoon dealt with the emotional flare-ups we could expect in the months ahead.

"Anger, lethargy, discouragement, depression—these are all part of the body's vigorous efforts to detoxify itself," he warned. "They can begin at any time. Some start a few days into the therapy while others may not appear for several weeks, but the first are usually the worst."

I thought of the ten-day rage Beata said she had experienced during her three-week stay at the clinic. That was one flare-up I should be spared, I thought. Having grown up with a father whose temper was constantly on the boil, I had learned early on how to keep my own anger firmly battened down.

I was sitting next to Pearl, whose gum-chewing asides I was trying to ignore, while on my right was an elderly gentleman I had seen walking in the corridor upstairs. A tall gaunt figure, he would take a few steps, stop, and breathe heavily before shuffling on.

"… And now," Frye was saying, turning to the subject of the environment, "most of the world's topsoil is gone, washed into the sea as a result of our mismanagement of earth's limited resources—" He stopped suddenly, for an unpleasant odor had entered the room.

"Jesus!" croaked Pearl. "What's that smell?" We glanced out the window where a man with a tank on his back was spraying around the building. "Ye gods!" shrieked Pearl, "it's pesticides!"

A strangled sound on my right made me turn.

"I've got to get out of here," gasped the old man. "I have lung cancer…. I can't take this."

"Neither can I!" I said, as my own lungs began to constrict. "Let's go!"

I took his arm and we headed toward the door, Frye's lecture forgotten in the ensuing consternation. Mounting the stairs as fast as his legs and lungs would allow, we finally reached the old man's room. There he hooked himself up to an oxygen tank that stood in the corner. I waited until his breathing had eased before returning to my room. By then I, too, was in need of some oxygen. A cylinder should have been in the hall, but it had disappeared, so I rang for another one.

When it arrived, the plastic mask smelled so strongly of polyvinyl chloride that any benefit gained from the oxygen was vitiated by the odor of the outgassing chemical. The masks in the ECU had been ceramic and the hose made of odorless polyurethane tubing.

By dinnertime I was sufficiently recovered to descend to the dining room, only to find the annex, too, had been sprayed. What madness had overtaken this clinic? I wondered. How could Charlotte *allow* such poisons to be used near patients who were so ill?

"Do you know what that stuff was they sprayed here today?" asked Randy, whose appearance at dinner that evening was a heartening surprise. "It was malathion. I recognized it 'cause we've used it on the farm."

"But malathion is supposed to be safe," said Morris.

"Not for people with cancer it's not safe," said Randy. "They've been spraying the kitchen, too, so now all our good organic food is probably contaminated as well. Hell!" he said, throwing down his napkin in disgust. "This whole damned place is contaminated! I'm going to have my dinner sent to my room."

He rose, and leaning heavily on his wife's arm, made his way out of the room. I left soon after, since my breathing had become labored again and my hands were bright red. *What in the name of Heaven are we doing to the planet?* I wondered. *What in God's name are we doing to ourselves?*

Half a century ago, Rachel Carson warned us about malathion:

> The alleged "safety" of malathion rests on rather precarious ground, although—as often happens—this was not discovered until the chemical had been in use for several years. Malathion is "safe" only because the mammalian liver, an organ with extraordinary protective power, renders it relatively harmless. The detoxification is accomplished by one of the enzymes of the liver. If, however, something destroys this enzyme or interferes with its action, the person exposed to malathion receives the full force of the poison. Unfortunately for all of us, opportunities for this sort of thing to happen are legion. A few years ago a team of Food and Drug Administration scientists discovered that when malathion and certain other organic phosphates are administered simultaneously, a massive poisoning results—up to fifty times as severe as would be predicted on the basis of adding together the toxicities of the two. In other words, one-hundredth of the lethal dose of each compound may be fatal when the two are combined.

The malathion exposure had set me back a week in the therapy. Panic attacks, hypersensitivity, exhaustion—all had returned, and my hair looked as though I had just seen a ghost. Dismayed at this setback, I wondered what Gerson had to say about pesticides in his book:

> … Pesticide and herbicide spraying anywhere near the home is devastating to the healthy body, much more to the debilitated healing body. Equally toxic is water pollution with fluorides, herbicides, pesticides, nitrates, silica and arsenic, etc. The patient cannot heal properly if the body continues to be contaminated.

The next morning, I looked in on the old man to see how he had weathered the exposure. He was sitting listlessly in his chair.

"I'm still having respiratory problems," he said, "although my primary cancer is in the prostate. My back has been hurting me something terrible, too, but that's probably because of my job."

"Oh? What do you do?"

"I'm a carpet cleaner by profession, but for the last few months I've been laying carpets—been down on my hands and knees a lot, you know, bending over."

I gasped. Not only had this gentle man been breathing the chemicals from carpets and underlay for years, he had been inhaling their toxic vapors for months at close range! I thought back to the day wall-to-wall carpeting was installed in my new flat, and the devastating illness that had felled me that same night.

"Have you ever considered," I asked carefully, "that your cancer might have been caused by the chemicals you have worked with for years? The chemicals that outgas from carpeting, I mean."

"Why no," he said. "It's never occurred to me."

I looked into his kind, trusting eyes and wanted to weep for his innocence. Would the day ever come when new carpets carried a government health warning?

BEWARE!
THE CHEMICALS IN THIS CARPET CAN BE
HAZARDOUS TO YOUR HEALTH!

When Charlotte came by the next day, I began to tell her about the malathion, but she had already been briefed.

"That *never* should have happened," she said angrily. "But you see, the Mexican government has a law that all public buildings and private institutions must be sprayed once a month."

"Once a month! But that's insane!"

"Of course it is. Which is why we've had 'an arrangement' to ensure that no spraying is done inside our front gate. Something must have gone wrong yesterday. I'm terribly sorry. But I should explain that I'm not in control here. I don't own the clinic."

"You don't? I thought you did."

"No, it's owned by the Mexican doctors who run it. Foreigners aren't allowed to have a clinic in Mexico, unless it's owned by Mexicans. They don't give us the same privileges here that we give them in our country. My position here is only an advisory one. I can suggest, but I cannot enforce."

Then that explained the shambolic approach to hygiene I had observed, such as the closet door I never saw closed though it bore the sign: *POR FAVOR MANTENIR CERRADA LA PUERTA; QUARTA SEPTICO! (Please keep this door closed; septic area!)*

We discussed the prevailing ignorance of government agencies about the systemic effects of chemicals and their threat to human health.

"Almost everyone we see here who is suffering from motor neuron disease has had insecticide poisoning," said Charlotte. That's what insecticides are—neurotoxins."

"Motor neuron disease?"

"That's amyotrophic lateral sclerosis, or ALS," she explained, "better known as Lou Gehrig's disease. Sprays and inhaled toxins damage the brain and cause the motor neurons to malfunction. They also cause mental and emotional problems, including depression."

Her mention of ALS reminded me of the woman in a wheelchair I had seen for the first time at lunch that day. Unable to talk or do anything for herself, she was being fed by a paid caregiver, her face a study in frustration. If she needed something, all she could do was move her eyes in anguished entreaty, hoping her caregiver would be watching and could interpret her meaning.

I mentioned her plight to Charlotte, in part because I wondered what the woman was doing at the clinic.

"I doubt we can do much for her at this stage," said Charlotte. "Motor neuron disease is one of the worst things that can happen to a person. Melanoma? A *cinch* to cure by comparison. Give me a simple melanoma any day! What makes ALS so tragic is that the peripheral motor nerves and the muscles waste away, while the mind remains clear to the end. Body and brain stop communicating. You can't move, you can't speak, and eventually you can't even swallow. Each day you lose more control over your body—a body in which the mind remains trapped—until you finally choke to death. Compared with ALS, cancer is a snap, believe me!"

I thought again of that insecticide spray gun I had used so wantonly against a few bugs, inhaling its toxic vapors for hours afterward in a sealed room. The thought of how easily I might have developed ALS instead of pan-sensitivity sent a shiver of fear through me, like the aftershock of a narrow escape. To be imprisoned in the body, unable to speak or read or do anything for oneself; to be dependent on others for the rest of one's life and condemned to a slow, agonizing death.... Compared to that sort of torment, I, too, would prefer cancer, *any* affliction that would allow me at least to communicate—even if all I had to communicate was my despair.

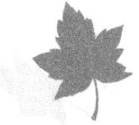

CHAPTER TWENTY-TWO

The pastor's proximity was becoming bothersome. Like a musical toothache, his guitar throbbed in the corridor, when he wasn't playing a tape of one of his sermons through a portable speaker. Did the man never pray silently to his God? Is the Lord so deaf He hears us only when we shout? In England, they used to say the landed gentry sent the fool of the family into the church. In America, the failed pop singer goes into evangelism.

One morning, when I had reached the end of my frail tether, I decided to confront Jimmy and plead for some Christian mercy. Striding into his room, I found him stretched out on the bed in jeans and a striped T-shirt, practicing the passage that had me climbing the wall for the past twenty minutes. Roy was in the bathroom taking a shower.

"Jimmy," I began, "could you *please* play your guitar somewhere else? I love music, but when I need to work, it shatters my concentration. I assure you that if *you* were the patient here, and something I did was disturbing *you*, I would desist."

He gave me a long, penetrating look, before placing his guitar on the floor. Then, folding his hands, he recited a passage from scripture: "Whoever having this world's good and seeing his brother hath need, shutteth not up his bowels of compassion."

"Why thank you, Jimmy," I said, disarmed. "I appreciate that, I really do."

"That's okay," he said. "While you were talking, the Lord spoke to me and said that I should do whatever I could to help a sister in need."

"Well, that's very generous of you," I said, envying his hotline to God. Roy emerged from the bathroom wearing a blue bathrobe and towel-drying his hair. "By the way, Jimmy, I've been meaning to ask you: how have you been able to take time away from your ministry to accompany Roy here? After all, he doesn't appear to need a caregiver, any more than I do."

"I came," said Jimmy solemnly, "because Jesus told me to, to support a brother."

For a moment I wondered what had come over Jesus, sending Jimmy to try my soul, when he should have been healing the lame and the sick.

Suddenly, he asked, "Are you a practicing Christian?"

The question caught me off guard. Aware that we were on delicate ground, I chose my words with care.

"I think I'm trying to be a practicing human being, but if you mean do I have a specific religion, the answer is no—though I used to be a Christian Scientist."

"Oh, well then," he said, "you weren't really a Christian; Christian Science is just a cult."

Surprised at this view, I asked Jimmy how he had arrived at that assessment. He reached for one of the leaflets on his nightstand and presented it to me. A church handout, it contained potted histories of four religions it claimed were doing the work of the devil—Christian Science being one. Intrigued, I read its description of the faith I had followed for thirty-five years.

"I'm afraid, Jimmy," I said, returning the leaflet to him, "that whoever wrote this has got the wrong end of the stick. If they had done their homework, they would know that far from doing the work of the devil, Christian Science denies the very existence of that personage."

It had been foolish to reply, of course; debates about religion are invariably futile. I would have enjoyed telling Jimmy about the poltergeist in our London flat and things that went bump in the night and invisible energy lines that answered to color and were found with a forked stick. If it was the devil and his works Jimmy was after, I could do him better than Christian Science. But he was trawling for souls, and mine was clearly ripe for redemption.

"It's still just a cult," he said. "There's only one true faith and unless you become reconciled to God in the name of Jesus Christ and accept the Lord Jesus as your Savior...."

"Forgive me, Jimmy," I interrupted, "but it *is* possible to have an abiding faith without having a religion."

"Without religion you can't be saved," he said, sternly. "Man is a sinner and needs to be saved. The Bible tells us so."

"Be that as it may," I nattered on, "although there is much good in most religions, there is also so much bigotry and hate in some that 'I prefer to be a sect by myself,' as Thomas Jefferson said. After all," I added, shamelessly showing off all those years of Bible study, "What does the Lord require of thee, but to do justly, and to love mercy, and to walk humbly with thy God?" *(Micah 6:8)*

A look of infinite pity spread over Jimmy's face. Undaunted, I waffled on, resorting to the familiar metaphor of the mountain we're all climbing, though taking different paths, and that as long as we meet at the top.... But I could see from his face that my little homily was in no way getting me off the hook.

"Well," I concluded, a touch cravenly, "at least I'm not an atheist or an agnostic."

"In that case," he said, "I will pray for you. I will pray that you return to Jesus."

"Thank you, Jimmy. I'm not sure I ever left him, but I can use all the prayers you've got."

On this note of conciliation, if not agreement, I returned to my room, Roy having remained mute the while.

Later, wondering what it was about the fundamentalists that I found so irksome, I decided it was their awful sanctimony. The trouble with born-again Christians was that they were even more tiresome the second time around.

There was something pitiless and hard in the belief that God speaks only to one group of people, while condemning the rest to eternal perdition. Wouldn't a loving Father want *all* His children to be saved, the lost sheep above all? If there really were but one true faith, surely the millions who have been seeking it for millennia would have reached some consensus by now, instead of blowing each other to bits in sectarian wars.

At lunch the next day, Charlotte shared with us one of the problems the institute was facing at that time.

"The biggest problem is finding doctors to train in the Gerson method since it's illegal in the US for them to treat cancer with nutrition. Even those doctors who've been cured by the therapy could lose their license if they recommend it to their patients."

Wearily, as if depleted by her long struggle to preserve her father's legacy, Charlotte added: "Little has changed since my father's day, when *JAMA* rejected every article he submitted for fear of losing its pharmaceutical advertisers. How could the journal give space to a doctor who cured cancer without drugs? What would become of the billion-dollar cancer research industry? It would be put out of business, that's what, since its business consists of research for more drugs."

Charlotte's comments have grown even more apposite since 1985. Indeed, the "cure for cancer" is like the Second Coming. We are told it is imminent, we are waiting for it to happen, but if it appears in a form different from the one we expect, we reject it. And crucify it.

We have more freedom of religion in America than we do freedom of medical choice. Any charismatic con man can proclaim "God has told me that ..." and establish a church that rakes in millions of tax-free dollars, but a doctor who cures cancer without drugs is left to the dubious mercies of a medical theocracy.

Hal was not in the dining room that day, so I stopped by his room after lunch and was surprised to find him packing to go home.

"But how will you manage the long trip to Australia, Hal?" I asked, wondering how he would manage the drive to the airport. "Won't that be a grueling trip?"

"Yes, but I have to go. I've run out of money and besides, I don't think the therapy is helping me. I just want to go home and be with my family."

I longed to say, "Get thee to hospice," but didn't know if Australia had a hospice movement. Instead, hoping to give him a chuckle, I told him about my talk with J.J. and the discovery that what I thought was my former faith was actually a cult.

Far from being amused, Hal took up where Jimmy left off, and I found myself being hectored by a Seventh Day Adventist. Seizing his Bible, Hall cited chapter and verse in support of Adventist belief. As far as I could make out, is based on "the seven Cs," Christ being the first, the cross the second—and I've forgotten the rest.

"We go to church on Saturday instead of Sunday," Hal explained, "Saturday being the seventh day of the calendar, which is where our name comes from. And we believe The Second Coming is imminent. When you die," he added with rising fervor, "if you're a Christian, you'll be at peace when you join Christ in His heavenly mansion for a thousand years. The Christian dead will be the first to rise. All others will stay in the ground during the thousand years while Satan roams the earth with his evil angels, trying to convert those who remain.

"None of your reincarnation rubbish!" he snorted, referring to a remark I had let fall during a previous visit.

Apparently, a thousand years in the heavenly mansion were preferable to an afterlife in which the mistakes made in this one might be redeemed in the next. What happened to the Christian dead when the thousand years were up I wondered? Were they turfed out of the mansion or could the lease be renewed? Prudence kept me from asking, for there was no warmth in Hal's philippic, no hint of humor or scintilla of doubt. And "without the saving grace of doubt," wrote Frances Wickes, "man never arrives at the faith which is his own."[1]

1 *The Inner World of Choice*

By the time I bade Hal goodbye, I was so God-smacked I felt the whole world could do with a radical theodectomy. It had been a long time since I'd encountered so much rigidity of belief—rigidity in the sense of clinging passionately to something, whether the thing clung to is right or wrong. A bit of therapeutic blasphemy would be no bad thing, I conjectured. God can take it, even if some of His children can't.

But then, maybe Hal was having a flare-up.

On the way back to my room, I was reminded of the Buddhist story about God and Satan, who were walking together one day when they saw a man some distance ahead bend down and pick up something that glowed brightly in his hand. On seeing this, Satan gave a cry of delight.

Puzzled, God asked what had pleased him so.

"That man has just found a piece of the truth," replied Satan.

"But why should that make you happy?" asked God.

"Because now he's going to *organize* it!" grinned Satan.

The more fervently the agents of God tried to hector me into holiness, the more I gave thanks for the Founding Fathers, who, when they framed the Constitution, took care to ensure not only our freedom *of* religion, but our freedom *from* religion as well.

As E. B. White observed:

> Democracy is itself a religious faith, for some it comes close
> to being the only formal religion they have. And so when I
> see the first faint shadow of orthodoxy sweep across the sky,
> feel the first cold whiff of its blinding fog steal in from the sea,
> I tremble all over, as though I had just seen an eagle go by,
> carrying a baby.

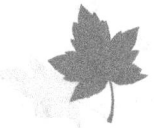

CHAPTER TWENTY-THREE

I had run out of batteries for my tape recorder. Told they could be found at *La Bottica*, one of several small shops across the street from the clinic, I set out to explore the amenities that lay beyond our oasis. Dodging the exhaust fumes of a passing car, I reached the shops that stood like a hyphen between an old warehouse at one end and a PE-MEX petrol station-*cum*-garage at the other. Large faded letters on the roof of the warehouse spelled, *LAMINA DE ASBESTOS.*

I found the batteries (Duracell® look-alikes that went dead after three days), then poked my nose into the adjoining shops—a liquor store, a clothing store, and an all-purpose store that sold, among other things, chile rellenos, jars of mole and adobo sauces, fried chicken wrapped in banana leaves, and other comestibles that would have given Dr. Gerson heartburn in his grave.

Not far from the shops a vendor was hawking chunks of gray meat bubbling in a vat of stomach-turning oil. It seemed ironic that Gerson's therapy had to take refuge in a country that ignored every principle upon which it was based.

A cement wall stood between the last store and the warehouse with an opening that proved too tempting to resist. I stepped through it and found large sheets of asbestos stacked on either side, their flaking corners accessible to the fingers of any inquisitive child. What a reckless country this is! I thought—storing crumbling asbestos mere yards from where food and drink are being consumed.

How many fibers had drifted over the road to La Gloria? I wondered. How many patients, arriving with terminal cancer, went home with a little more asbestos in their lungs?

In his 1987 book, *High-Tech Holocaust,* James Bellini observed:

In North America the old, developed world rubs shoulders with the newly industrialized; the first generation of acid polluters co-exists alongside one of the newest entrants to the league of contaminators. And it is the rise of younger economies such as Mexico, with their passion for development and lower regard for regulatory controls, that threatens to turn an already unacceptable level of world-wide acidity—the accumulated dross of a century of profligate old world frenzy—into a truly global eco-disaster.

Returning to the clinic, I found its own depredations continuing apace. As I climbed the stairs, I passed a languorous worker stripping paint from the iron banister with a chemical that smelled suspiciously like creosote. He was still at it when I went down to dinner, holding my nose as I hurried past him to avoid the fumes.

To my dismay, the floor of the administration building was covered with an odiferous foam, the smell of which had spread into the dining room as well. The true miracle of this place, I decided, was not that it cured cancer, but that it cured it in *spite* of environmental ignorance on a monumental scale.

I was recording the day's events in my diary the following afternoon, when a commotion in the corridor drew me away from my desk. On opening my door I saw chairs being arranged against the wall and a gray-haired "gringo" positioning a group of children for some sort of performance.

"That's Dr. Long," explained a patient. "He's an American. He teaches music at a religious mission in San Diego and comes to Mexico every Friday to give music lessons to the children. Once a month he brings them here to sing for us."

Delighted that my stay coincided with this event, I took a chair and was soon transported by the children's sweet, piping voices singing their native songs. Bright, upraised eyes followed their leader's hands as he varied the *tempi,* with a sweep of his arms here, a raised palm there, or a finger pressed to his lips for a final *pianissimo.*

Suddenly, the thrum of a guitar made me twist around in my seat. There framed in the doorway stood Jimmy, guitar strap slung over his shoulder, head bobbing in time with the music, contributing a few superfluous riffs of his own. When the concert ended he stepped forward and made a little speech of thanks on behalf of us all, bestowing upon the older man and his charges a blessing that would not have disgraced the Pope.

Two nights later, I lay in bed listening to the muffled sounds in the next room—voices laughing, drawers being opened and shut, and objects being dragged across the floor. My neighbors, I had learned, would be decamping in the morning.

"*Adios,* Jimmy," I murmured, sliding happily under the covers. "*Vaya con Dios.*"

Like everything else at La Gloria, the telephone system was capricious. With the end of my stay approaching, I'd been trying to reach my daughter Amy, who was supposed to meet me at the San Diego airport on the seventeenth and drive me to Los Angeles for my flight back to London. I finally got through to her on the sixteenth to let her know that a car would be taking me over the border early in the morning, and the approximate time of my arrival.

That afternoon, Dr. Melendez came to discuss the food I would be taking with me on the flight home the next day. Seeing me exhausted in bed, she said, "Do not worry that you are feeling tired. The exhaustion is a sign of the healing process as the toxins begin to enter your bloodstream."

"My only fear is of having a flare-up on the plane," I said, "when I won't be able to detoxify for fifteen hours or more."

"Some flare-ups don't start until the fourth or fifth week," said Dr. Melendez, in a failed attempt to reassure me.

"But how will I know when I'm having a flare-up in London if it's a sign that I'm getting better or a sign that I'm getting worse?" I asked, anxiously.

"You will know," she said, "your body will tell you. Now, for the trip home you will have a thermos of soup, one of tea, one of carrot juice, and two baked potatoes. The car will be here at 7:00 in the morning. You will let me know about your progress when you return home, yes?"

"Oh, if only I could take you with me," I said, flinging my arms around her and feeling less confident than ever about the months ahead.

"I've just learned that Jaquie Davison has dyed her dark hair blonde again," said Charlotte, during her final visit that afternoon, "even though she knows how dangerous hair dye is for those who've had cancer."

Foolish Jaquie, I thought; so much for "keeping our temple clean." It did make me wonder, though, about some of the people God saves, compared to so many of those whom He lets die. To Charlotte, I said,

"It seems she had the experience, but missed the meaning."

"She's crazy," shrugged Charlotte.

I would be leaving at seven the next morning, so I said my goodbyes at dinner. There were only a few remaining patients with whom I'd spent much time. Hal had returned to Australia—safely, I hoped—and Pearl had taken her husband home to Ohio. Morris would be staying on, of course, but Tina's future was uncertain. Indeed, some months after my return to London, I heard that she had died. As for Randy, my inner soothsayer could only weep for him and his family.

I had been feeling off-color all afternoon; not ill, exactly, but unaccountably anxious and on edge. While packing that evening, a cloud of depression descended over me like a shroud. I couldn't think why. I wasn't sad about leaving; on the contrary, I couldn't wait to get home. I *was* concerned about the flight, but I had put some emergency supplies in a carry-on, chiefly for the sense of security they gave me. Why, then, this mounting anxiety, this nameless pressure bearing down on my spirit?

By half past ten, my heart was racing and a tiny motor seemed to be pulsing in the ball of each foot. The symptoms were similar to those I felt when being affected by a fractured energy line, only stronger. How could this be? I had dowsed the room before leaving the annex and it had dowsed clear.

The return of a sensitivity I had all but forgotten for three weeks was worrying. I took out my Y-rod and explored the room again, but it still dowsed quiet. Mistrusting the response, I picked up the color wheel and instantly the rod went berserk, twisting and flipping over in my hands so uncontrollably I could hardly keep hold of it. The whole room was a kaleidoscope of fractured energy lines. What on earth could be causing this aberration? These energies weren't here before, or I would have felt them.

A sudden panic gripped me as I realized that even here my condition was beyond help or understanding. With mounting anxiety I prayed, *Please, God, spare me this trial on the flight home!*

The night ahead loomed as dread-filled as all those other nights I thought I had left behind in London. Toward midnight, my body went into overdrive: my feet throbbed, my fingers pulsed, and my heart thumped wildly in my chest. I sought relief with the oxygen tank. It was still in my room, though it shouldn't have been. It made no difference. My last coffee break had been at ten. I took another. I drank some chamomile tea. I lay down, longing for sleep, but my heart beat so heavily when I was prone I had to get up. Only if I kept moving could I keep these energies from piercing through me like laser beams.

By midnight, my teeth were on edge and my scalp felt as though it was crawling with maggots. I washed my hair. At half past one I took another coffee break. It was no use. Whatever this was, the therapy couldn't handle it.

I must have dropped off from exhaustion around 3:00 a.m., for when I woke at 5:00, I realized I had fallen asleep. I got up to go to the bathroom and glanced in the mirror—then stared in disbelief at my reflection. The curl had returned to my hair! It was as wavy as it had been in its crowning glory days. If this was a sign, I thought, it was one I would cling to in the months ahead.

Amy was waiting for me as my car pulled up at the airport. We embraced, and with her strong young arms around me, I felt reconnected to the world, after my sojourn in the land of carrot juice and cancer.

We set off for Los Angeles in her car and now that my body was in motion again, my symptoms began to recede. By the time we reached LAX they were almost gone, and I no longer needed to hide my hair with a head scarf.

Sitting with my daughter in the departure lounge, chatting about things that had nothing to do with the body and its ills, I began to feel like a normal human being again. I had forgotten how hostile public places could be until the smoke-filled air reached my sinuses and I felt a headache coming on.

Amy had to leave before my flight was called, and as we hugged goodbye a great loneliness welled up inside me. Would I be able to return next year to see my father and daughters again? Would I be well enough to go anywhere while doing the therapy? A steel clamp seemed to be tightening around my skull, and a nasty flare-up was looming. It had been eight hours since the last detox coffee break and my body was on a four-hour schedule. If it got worse on the plane....

Desperate times call for desperate measures. I grabbed my carry-on, fetched some coffee from the dispenser in the lounge, topped it up with tap water in the Ladies', and locked myself in the loo for the disabled. So what if the coffee wasn't organic or the water distilled?

The procedure was under way when someone entered the room. I lay very still, praying she would not be disabled. Instead of using the facilities, however, she just stood there—doing what, I wondered; putting on full makeup, apparently, from the sound of things. I heard the click of a purse opening and objects being set down on the counter, followed by long stretches of agonizing silence in between. *Oh go,* I prayed, *please go! What's taking you so long?*

At length, I heard her gathering up her things, followed by the sound of the door opening and the slow, sucking noise as it closed on her retreating footsteps. With a sigh of relief, I completed the operation and returned to the lounge. Even before my flight was called, the headache lifted.

We had been airborne for less than an hour when my hair began to wilt again, its brief glory undone by the cabin's recycled air. With a heavy heart, I reached for the hated head scarf. I should have known the miracle was too good to last.

An hour later my headache returned—this time with such a blinding vengeance I wanted to hurl myself out of the plane. There was no way I could endure ten more hours of this agony or even ten more minutes. I staggered up the aisle and found a flight attendant in the galley. After confiding my predicament to her I asked, "So is there a loo on the plane a bit larger than the one in business class?" If the attendant thought me mad or my needs bizarre, she didn't let on.

"The one on the upper deck is slightly bigger," she said, pouring some coffee into a mug and handing it to me, "although not by much, I'm afraid."

I thanked her, and with the mug in one hand, my carry-on in the other, I climbed the stairs to the deck above. The film had just started, so with luck I wouldn't be disturbed. I spread my trousers on the floor, adopted a tight fetal position, and by the grace of God and Gerson, achieved the impossible. Soon afterwards, my headache was gone— this time for good—and I spent the rest of the flight in relative comfort.

Albert Schweitzer was right: Max Gerson *was* a medical genius. He was also, on this particular occasion, my savior in absentia.

Three weeks later, after the therapy had been ticking over in London, I wrote to Charlotte:

"Am I the first Gerson person to have negotiated a coffee break at 35,000 feet over the Atlantic?"

Her reply cut me down to size.

"Sorry," she wrote back, "another patient has beaten you to it."

Ah, well, the suffering I was spared that day was worth more than any entry in a Gerson Book of Records. Recalling the high-flying headaches I had endured in the past, I could only bless the doctor who had saved me from what would have been the most agonizing journey of my life.

Max Gerson could not have imagined the lengths to which some of his patients would take his therapy in extremis. Yet such radical improvisation was no more than an extension of what we had learned at the clinic, what Gerson himself preached in his book: namely, the importance of keeping the body detoxified—and, above all, the *vital* importance of taking responsibility for our own health.

CHAPTER TWENTY-FOUR

My first week home was hectic, trying to maintain the rhythm of juices, meals, and enemas, while teaching the therapy's mechanics to Isilda, the Portuguese helper I had engaged. Isilda proved to be an absolute treasure. At first. Unfortunately, I hadn't foreseen the hazards of adding to my quiet way of life the live-in presence of a forty-five-year-old Portuguese firebrand.

Short, squat, and tempestuous, she tackled the kitchen chores with a vigor that made up in zest for what it lacked in equanimity. Her take-charge efficiency was a godsend, since it freed me to work on the book I was trying to write about my adoptive experience.

Deaf to noise and a stranger to silence, she banged doors, ran the vacuum cleaner under my feet while I worked, and flung cutlery into the kitchen drawer with such a clatter it was a job holding my thoughts together. She was suspicious of all things mechanical and took an instant dislike to the Norwalk® juicing machine—a costly piece of equipment I had imported at some expense from the US. Dismissing the instruction book with a shrug, she jammed vegetables into the grinder with such vigor that bits and pieces wound up all over the ceiling and cupboard doors.

"It really is quite easy to keep this from happening, Isilda," I said, showing her for the nth time how to keep the housing covered during the grinding process. But Isilda and sweet reason were not on speaking terms.

"I do how you say," she replied irritably, "but the ve-ge-tables—they no like to stay in!"

It says much for the Norwalk's construction that it withstood twelve months of Isilda's abuse, while churning out the enzyme-rich juices on which the therapy relied. I did, however, sympathize with her complaints about having to make ten juices a day—actually it should have been thirteen, but she *had* been warned.

Marching up to my desk with a glass of carrot juice, she would set it down as though it was hemlock, saying, "I tell you this, my dear—all this juices is no good for your kidneys!" She was equally disapproving of the salt-free, sugar-free, meat-free, organic meals she had to prepare.

"How you eat this food?" she demanded. "Is no taste! When I eat, make me sick!"

She was, of course, free to make for herself whatever her Portuguese palate preferred, but Isilda, I soon discovered, was one of life's grumblers. At first her tetchiness amused me, for she was so manifestly eager to help me get well—as long as her help could be given in a way that *she* could understand.

"Tell me how I can *help* you!" she would cry over my prostrate form, when I was feeling too ill almost to speak. All I wanted from Isilda—all I needed from her—was a steady supply of juices and her support for what I was doing, whether she approved of it or not.

Convinced the therapy was making me worse, she would stand by my bedridden form, arms akimbo on her sturdy hips and say, "This thing you do—I no understand. I see you are in pain. You say, 'That is good.' When *I* have pain that is *not* good. It tell me something wrong. When you are sick, you say, 'That is good.' When you are *more* sick, 'That is better?' Is crazy therapy!"

"Yes, well, could we discuss it some other time, Isilda? Just give me until January and we'll see who's winning, the therapy or the pain."

At this, she would march out of the room, arms brushing the sides of her apron in that gesture I came to know meant it was *my* loss if I ignored her good advice.

On September 19, a huge earthquake hit Mexico City, a staggering 8.1 on the Richter scale. As I read of the widespread damage and loss of life, I was grateful the clinic was far enough away to have been spared.

My first healing flare-ups in London were mild. A toe I had broken several times began to swell, painful calluses appeared on the balls of my feet, and the skin on my fingers began to peel away in ever-widening circles. Arrhythmic heartbeats returned, as did that sick-all-over-feeling in the morning. Now, however, I understood—or rather, accepted on faith—that these were proofs the detoxification process was underway. There were times when faith in Gerson had to be stronger than faith in God.

One day, when my fingers suddenly went numb, save for a faint tingling at the tips, I grew alarmed, because I'd heard this was a symptom—a precursor of multiple sclerosis. During one such episode, I turned to the chapter on insecticides in Gerson's book and read:

> Areas of skin become exquisitely hypersensitive ... or irregular numbness, tingling sensations, itching or crawling sensations, or a feeling of localized heat may take place.

Further on, referring to experiments with insecticides conducted by the FDA as long ago as the 1940s, he wrote:

> F.D.A. scientists have also shown that it is possible to store many times the amount in the body-fat that would be acutely fatal intravenously in a single dose.... Cumulative intoxication from extremely small amounts in food can thus be as dangerous as direct exposure to much larger amounts.

It was to hasten the exit of these cumulative toxins that Gerson added coffee enemas to his regime. "Patients have to know," he wrote, "that the coffee enemas are not given for the function of the intestines but for the stimulation of the liver."

A flyer arrived in the mail one day inviting me, in exuberant type, to *SKIP OVER HOT COALS TO CONQUER YOUR FEAR!*—the same exercise Frye had recommended to us at the clinic. Designed apparently for the pain-deprived, it promised to confer courage at the risk of a slight burn on the soles of one's feet:

> This course enables people to transcend fear, to discover latent powers, do the seemingly impossible and use these skills in other areas of life.

I tossed it into the wastebasket. Been there, doing that now.

In London, organic vegetables were imported, expensive, and in short supply. The only sources available in 1985 were a Whole Foods store on Baker Street and a supplier in Covent Garden—an amiable young bandit, Ken, who shamelessly exploited our dependence on him for organic produce. Occasionally, he would slip a non-organic item into my order, on the reasonable assumption that I wouldn't notice the difference. My body did, though, and alerted me to the impostor soon after it was consumed. Eventually, I found an honest greengrocer in Chelsea, an Indian, whose few organic vegetables, imported from Germany, were displayed in their original cartons, marked *Biologique.*

Four weeks into the therapy my body went suddenly into overdrive. My feet throbbed, my hair went limp, and my heart began to do its funny dance. Wondering what the cause could be, I remembered we had run out of organic carrots the day before, and to tide us over until Ken's delivery, I had bought five pounds of carrots at the supermarket.

Following a hunch, I went to the kitchen where Isilda was preparing dinner.

"Isilda," I asked, "when did you start using the new carrots?"

"This afternoon, last two juices. Why?"

"No reason," I said, dodging a sermon. "I just wondered."

Clever body, I thought. You knew, I didn't.

I had been reading *Silent Spring* again and found this paragraph in my well-thumbed copy:

> Carrots absorb more insecticide than any other crop studied; if the chemical used happens to be lindane, carrots actually accumulate higher concentrations than are present in the soil.

Had Rachel Carson not died so tragically young from breast cancer, she might have added the more recent discovery that when commercial carrots are juiced, the pesticides become more concentrated in the juice. One assumes this applies to all non-organic vegetables and fruits.

Meanwhile, Isilda's caregiving, which at first had been such a comfort, was beginning to feel more like a cross. Occasionally, when I was having a flare-up, I had to conceal from her how ill I really felt if I wanted to avoid one of her lectures about the therapy. If she found me in mid-enema on the bathroom floor, she would stand in the doorway, all bossy briskness, and say, "I tell you this—all this enemas is no good for your behind!" Or, "I tell you this my dear—this therapy you do, it make you crackers!"

Notwithstanding her disapproval, Isilda kept the juices coming, and with the regime now in full swing, I was surprised at how well I had adapted to its restraints. Averse to commitment, and quickly bored with routine, I had embraced both as the price I had to pay for a restored immune system. My only fear was of having a flare-up the therapy couldn't handle—like the one that last night at the clinic, for if Gerson should fail, what then?

Only once did I weaken and break the rules. At the health food store one day, I lusted after a carob-coated rice cake. Well, rice was safe, wasn't it? And carob better than chocolate? So I bought two and ate them both on the spot.

Within minutes, my hands turned red and my throat seized up. *That's me,* I moaned, *the unteachable self-punisher!* Why did I think I could put something over on my body? It was so much wiser than I, and so vengeful. Stricken with shame, I fancied I could hear Dr. Gerson's voice scolding me from his perch in the pantheon:

"Well, if you don't stick to the rules, you deserve everything recidivism can throw at you."

Forgive me, Max. It won't happen again, I promise!

Locked as I now was into my salt-free, sugar-free, fat-free, dairy-free diet, all my gustatory pleasures of the past were a receding memory. I had to remind myself that if the prize was a restored immune system, what did they matter, a couple of years out of my life? After all, it had taken more than two years for my immune system to collapse.

I still looked forward to my book at enema-time, although there were days when I was too sick to read and could only lie on the bathroom floor, wishing for death. During one such break I was so exhausted I fell asleep, waking to find a hose stuck up my bottom and a nasty crick in my neck.

Sometimes it seemed the therapy's sole purpose was to destroy my dignity and reduce my ego to ashes. All the things I had been spared as a child—enemas, castor oil, preoccupation with the body's least elegant functions—were now part of my daily routine. More than ever I was glad I had been raised as a Christian Scientist, since this had spared me all the drugs that are being pumped so promiscuously into children today. Had I been given even a fraction of these when young, my immune system would have collapsed when I was in my twenties instead of my forties.

There were moments when it frightened me to realize how alone I was in this venture—like a rookie pilot flying solo over uncharted territory, aware that if I crashed there would be no hope of rescue or survival. I didn't like to bother Beata too often with questions, for she had her own busy life to lead, and besides, our problems were not the same.

The only person I could turn to when faith was faltering was Charlotte, but she was a continent away and not always available. Yet when she *was* there, the mere sound of that strong, confident voice on the phone was enough to put the starch back in my spine and renew my resolve. Without her voice at the end of the line, I might not have had the will to go on. She gave me hope and perspective on moonless nights. She was my long-distance cheerleader—my lifeline to recovery.

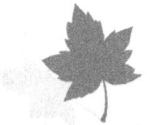

CHAPTER TWENTY-FIVE

October was a month of unremitting pain. Arthritis flared in every joint and aches in every muscle. When I tried to write, my fingers closed stiffly around the pen—and my neck, which I had injured when young, felt like a column of splintered glass. One night I reached for the primer and turned to the chapter on healing reactions:

> During the reaction, arthritic joints may become puffed up and more painful than previously experienced.

An understatement, certainly, but a reassuring one. How perverse to feel comforted from knowing that others have suffered in the same distressing way.

On the fourth of October, I decided to throw away all the antigen vaccines. It was an extravagant gesture, since they were expensive and I had used only half, but it seemed important to affirm my total reliance on the path I had chosen.

On the fifth, Beata rang to ask how I was getting on. After moaning to her about my arthritis, I moaned about my hair. I had already described its odd behavior that last night at the clinic and its subsequent relapse on the plane.

"And now it's gone all limp again!" I wailed.

"That's not possible," she said. "Hair is dead. It can't change. Its only life is in the roots."

"I know that, Beata. I can't understand either why mine acts so strangely—curling one day and collapsing the next—but it does. Do you think it's just a flare-up and therefore a good sign?"

"Well, everyone *I* know who has been on the therapy, their hair has got better, not worse, so I'm afraid it's not a very good sign."

Trust Beata to cheer me up, I thought. If only she weren't so honest.

Isilda's pep talks were worse. If I bewailed my thinning thatch she would say, "My hair, too, it go like that! Always change when I am nairvoos and upset!"

"But I'm only nervous and upset *because* my hair is falling out!" I would cry. Why did no one understand? If they couldn't see my hair was vanishing, it was only because I had so much to begin with.

When my allergies returned again in mid-October, I rang Beata.

"What can this mean?" I asked her.

"I've no idea," she said, "because no one I know has had your problem."

And that was my problem; none of the patients we knew had chemical poisoning, only cancer—although I was beginning to suspect a link between the two.

Other flare-ups occurred. Walking home from the Tube station one day, I suddenly doubled up with stabbing pains in the groin. Too worried to wait for a letter to creep through the post, I rang Charlotte as soon as I reached home.

"That's great!" she exclaimed. "A good sign the liver is beginning to get rid of its poisons."

I sighed. No wonder the therapy's dropout rate was high.

Meanwhile, Isilda's personality had been changing—from bossy but helpful, to stroppy and despotic. Having twigged by now that I was a wimp, she exploited my dependence upon her in earnest. Perhaps the juices were stressing her out, I reasoned, or maybe too much praise had gone to her head. If I said the slightest thing she could construe as critical, she would shrug and say, "You no like, I go!"

Too weak to stand up to her blackmail, and too easily intimidated, I resorted to craven appeasement, which only made her worse. St. Paul was wrong: The root of all evil is not the love of money, it's the love of *power!* Marching from the kitchen with juice in hand, Isilda would plonk it down on my desk, point to my typewriter and say, "You put in your book that I go to *Heaven* for making all this juices! My God, what a job!"

And so—very meekly—I put in my book: Isilda goes to heaven.

But she *had* been warned.

As the days stretched into weeks, and the weeks into months, I kept asking the same question: *Why does my body so mightily betray me?* I had never abused it, never even been tempted by the things today's youth can scarcely avoid, yet it was full of rebellion.

Gerson warns that cancer flare-ups can last from two to four days, and Beata recorded a total of twenty-eight flare-ups when she was doing the therapy. Being an arithmaphobe, I didn't even try to count mine, but they included migraine headaches, devastating fatigue, and days of such constant sneezing I seemed to be allergic to the universe. There was frustration with the functions that kept me body-bound and fury when their demands ate into my time for work. There were loneliness and doubt and fear that it might not work for me—that the map I'd been given to follow had been charted for a different journey.

"My, what a lot of Karma you must be working through!" remarked a new-age friend, who had been following my ups and downs with the therapy.

"Karma or chemicals," I retorted, "it is not a fun journey." Augusto Roa Bastos, described it best in *I, the Supreme*:

> I journeyed through all those great remotenesses with only my own person at my side, without anybody. Alone. Without family. Alone. Without anybody. Alone in a strange country,

the strangest one being that most my own. Alone. My trapped, lonely, alien country. Deserted. Alone. Full of my empty person.

Spot-on, Augusto.

And then there was depression—a full month of it. But I had a lot to be depressed about: losing my lovely hair, mistaking a terminal crisis for a healing flare-up, ending the therapy more sensitive than when I began, and so on. Frye warned us that depression was part of the healing process; he just forgot to add that it could be suicidal.

Thoughts of easeful death darkened many a midnight hour, the only deterrent being the fear of opting out of life before its purpose had been fulfilled—assuming it had one. What was I saving my life for anyway? I had achieved nothing, would never finish my book, would be missed by no one if I died—this last, perhaps, was a shade self-dramatizing.

There were times when I felt I couldn't go on, yet I couldn't go back. *You've come this far,* I told myself. *You can't stop now. But how long, oh Lord, how long?*

To my diary I whined: "Have I been trying to save my life, only to die—not in a paroxysm of pain, but in a whimper of despair?"

To this whimper of self-pity the only response was silence. Divine neglect, not divine punishment, is the worst.

Sometimes, the only thing that kept me going was hope—that, and telling myself that trials such as this afflict only the virtuous. Most of what sustains us in life is illusion, but is no less sustaining for that.

The word "courage" came often to mind, due to its irrelevance in hopeless situations. To be courageous requires the option *not* to be, such as taking a bullet in battle to save a comrade, or rescuing a drowning child when one hardly knows how to swim. Enduring what can't be escaped is not courage; it's fortitude.

In November, arthritic flare-ups were fewer, which suggested that some forms of arthritis might be caused by chemical deposits in the joints. If this is so, then the stiffening joint should be viewed as a warning to detoxify the body—not as a sign to add more chemicals in the form of drugs.

One morning I woke with my neck feeling like a block of crystal being crushed by a wrench. Pains were shooting through my legs, and my feet felt as though they were plugged into an electric socket. It was one of my strongest flare-ups to date, and the scariest. To be facing this crisis armed only with juices and enemas made me feel like a very small David confronting Goliath with an organic carrot. This Goliath, however, was a monster of many parts, all of them man-made, and all of them lethal.

Staggering to the bathroom, I glanced in the mirror—and recoiled from the face that stared back at me. I seemed to have morphed into some alien creature, my features distorted, my hair flying away in wisps from my head. I thought of the family friend who had contracted a mysterious disease while serving in the Pacific theater during World War II. Young and handsome when he left for the war, his features began to change before he was honorably discharged. His hair fell out, his body wasted away and he grew prematurely old before our eyes. When he died in his thirties, leaving a wife and young children, he was almost unrecognizable.

"Something he caught in the Pacific," the family said, but no one really knew.

Fortunately, my features soon returned to normal, but the incident gave me pause. Could that young soldier have been exposed to some unknown chemical in the 1940s? I knew a Vietnam War veteran who attributed the birth of an albino son, conceived after his return home, to his known exposure to Agent Orange. And I had met a group of Gulf War veterans whose afflictions were manifestly the result of some sort of chemical assault.

181

Perhaps the war to end all wars is being waged even now inside our bodies between the toxins we can neither see nor avoid, but whose cumulative power may one day bring us all down to defeat.

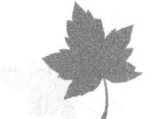

CHAPTER TWENTY-SIX

In November, my mastectomy scar began to itch, swell, and turn red. Could I be growing a new breast? I wondered. Alas, the therapy doesn't restore missing bits. Five days later the swelling was gone, leaving me in awe of the body's ability to tidy up the debris of an eleven-year-old operation.

I recalled my oncologist telling me that he wished all his patients were as easy as I was. At the time, I took this as a compliment. Now I knew that being "easy," being compliant, was precisely what I should *not* have been. I had yielded to the knife as trustingly as I had yielded to prayer, when what I should have done was rage, rebel, and refuse to be butchered. At least I'd had the wit to refuse the hysterectomy he wanted to perform—"to prevent your crazy hormones from creating cancer in the other breast," he explained. I had heard enough hysterectomy horror stories to know that when the time came, I wanted my menopause to be a natural one.

I thought of the so-called cancer-prone personality, suggested by Lawrence LeShan, whose books I was then reading. "Emotionally repressed, unable to express love or aggression," were two of the characteristics ascribed to such individuals. It was true I found it hard to express aggression, but emotionally repressed? Unable to express love? In my view, treating psychological traits as the cause of disease came dangerously close to blaming the victim.

Even Beata favored the psychological approach—understandably so, for by then she was a practicing psychotherapist.

One day, when we were discussing our different cancers, she proposed an exercise:

"Try to identify the psychological factors that might have contributed to the development of your cancer," she suggested.

I tried to do this, but truly could not see a connection between my psyche and a tumor growing in my breast. Even if there were one, what purpose could be served by identifying it? After all, we can't change our basic personalities. A more likely factor, I thought, would have been my father's cigars, which had made me a passive smoker for my first nineteen years of life.

Not that I denied the mind/body/spirit connection. How could I when members of my family and I myself had experienced numerous healings through Christian Science? All the same, I knew someone who fitted the cancer-prone personality to a "C," yet whom the disease had never touched, while others who did not conform to the pattern had nonetheless succumbed. Whatever psychological factors Beata felt had contributed to her cancer, it was still the body-bound Gerson Therapy that had cured her melanoma.

In November I received a letter from Nora, telling me of David's death.

"Even though it was expected," she wrote, "I'm still feeling devastated by his loss."

How hard it is, I reflected, when we are the ones left behind to believe that death is merely a change of worlds. Whatever view one holds of the hereafter—even if one holds none at all—life on this earth still unfolds through a veil of mystery.

By the tenth of November, I was detoxing so rapidly my body resembled a medical repertory company: *EACH DAY A NEW FLARE-UP! EACH WEEK A NEW CAST OF SYMPTOMS!* Some flare-ups were so strong I needed an extra coffee break at the intermission to clear them (I'd have settled for an intermission). Remissions were brief, however, and my body had only to dump more chemicals into my bloodstream for the parade of symptoms to resume its merry round. A frequent prayer at this time was *Dear God, get me through the night!*

As for my diary, what was I keeping a diary for? With no secrets to confide, no juicy scandals to record, mine was just a tedious record of symptoms, moans, and groans.

After one such crisis, I wrote to Charlotte, "What do they mean, these random pains—these hot flushes one moment, chills the next, and legs so weak I have to drag myself up the stairs?"

"We see that in patients who have old drug damage," she replied. "We always get a different reaction from the cancer patient, who usually hasn't been as totally pre-treated with drugs, unless they've had chemo. The drug damage and healing are rough."

So that was all right, then. Things were coming along nicely.

Seizing this small comfort, I soldiered on through an attack of cystitis, which mimicked one I'd had thirteen years earlier, and rashes that broke out on various parts of my body. By contrast, my swollen toe had returned to normal and as for the calluses on my feet, they were so nearly gone I could even forget about them during the day.

One morning, Isilda came to my room with a book in her hand.

"I like you read this book," she said. "If you do, it make you better."

A glance at the cover told me it was the Christian Science textbook, *Science and Health with Key to the Scriptures,* by Mary Baker Eddy.

"My friend, she take me to Wednesday night meeting," Isilda explained, "and I like very much. She give me tapes of sermons. I tell you, God will heal you if you read this book."

There was something endearing about the Catholic Isilda urging me to turn for help to the Protestant faith I had relinquished years before. I thanked her for her concern, told her I already had a copy of the book, and that I would read it again at the earliest opportunity.

On the seventeenth I felt an odd pressure in my lungs, similar to the one that occurred the day Clive left a malachite stone on my map. I called him to ask if this had happened again.

"No," he said. "In fact, I now keep your map in a manila envelope isolated from the others. Whatever is bothering you, the cause must be in your flat."

What could it be? I wondered.

Isilda was off that day, and I had managed to make only two juices. How anyone could do the therapy on their own, without help, was beyond me, yet I was told that a few plucky patients had done just that—and successfully, too.

I was in the kitchen that evening when Isilda returned around ten. As I went to greet her I caught a whiff of perfume. This surprised me, because she'd agreed not to use any scented products while living in the flat. In exchange for her compliance I supplied her with fragrance-free soap, hand lotion, and shampoo.

"Isilda," I asked, "are you wearing perfume?"

"I no wear perfume since I come here!" she said, crossly.

"But I can smell it, there's some sort of scent on your person."

"All I do—I put hair spray before I go out, that is all."

So *that's* what it was! The propellant in hair spray was one of the most volatile chemical pollutants. Isilda turned to go to her room, but I restrained her.

"Wait, Isilda, I know this is hard for you to understand, but for people who are chemically sensitive, *any* scented product can cause a reaction."

"But I put on and go right out!" she insisted, her face darkening.

"I understand that, but while *you* may have gone out, your hair spray stayed behind in the form of chlorofluorocarbons in the air."

She gave me a look of withering scorn. Isilda viewed my preoccupation with chemicals as the product of an addled brain. Yet she had told me that whenever a fly came near her she broke out in a rash. This seemed to me much odder than reacting to perfume. However, when a fly appeared in the flat one day, she did indeed develop a rash—even before she knew it was there. Like it or not, Isilda was every bit as freakish as I. Together, we proved that while you can fool the mind some of the time, you can't fool the body—at least, not for long.

Due to the sheer volume of vegetables the therapy required, I took Isilda with me when I went to the greengrocer's each week to help me carry them home. Striding ahead of me on the pavement, while I trailed behind her, like an untouchable, she cut a singular figure. Even poor Mr. Desai was not spared the sharp end of her tongue; her caustic comments about his blameless produce made me cringe with embarrassment.

"How do you put up with her?" he asked once, shaking his head after she had flounced out of the store while I was paying the bill.

"With difficulty," I sighed.

Three months into the therapy, I woke one morning with nausea, a crushing headache, and a body so stiff I had to ease it carefully out of bed. Turning once more to the primer's chapter on healing reactions, I read, "...Lack of appetite, nausea, headache, arthritic symptoms, flu-like aches in the body...."

Marginally less alarmed, I spent the day nursing my pounding head while trying to ignore Isilda's demands that I abandon "this therapy that make you more sick!"

That evening, while releasing an enema, a searing pain shot through my rectum—as though a hot poker had been thrust up my backside. The pain could not have lasted more than a minute, but it was so excruciating I cried out in agony. When it finally subsided, I searched the bowl for a sign of the cause. The only clue was the greenish color of the return, which meant that a strong detox phase was underway. Within an hour the headache and nausea were gone, and the stiffness, too, had eased by the next day.

No wonder Gerson patients say, "If you can survive the therapy, you can survive anything!"

But how could my body have harbored such a fiery substance un-awares—perhaps even for years? Could that have been the chemical that destroyed my eyelashes and eyebrows? Could it have been the acid I felt creeping under my scalp? Perhaps I had poisoned my hair follicles by dyeing my hair a more lively auburn. Charlotte warns cancer pa-tients not to dye their hair, because the scalp absorbs the chemical dyes through the pores. Oh, Charlotte, where were you when I was foolish and twenty? Where were you when I was foolish and forty!

Baffled by the burning backside incident, I rang Beata.

"Did anything like that happen to you when you were doing the therapy?" I asked.

"Not quite," she said, "but I once woke up with a bilious burning sensation in my mouth."

How strange. No wonder doctors scoffed at the idea of chemical sensitivity. What self-respecting physician would link a rectum on fire with pesticide poisoning or a bilious burning feeling in the mouth with melanoma die-off? Chemicals don't show up on their X-rays, ultrasounds, or CT scans. One has to know what to look for, and where—and how.

As evidence grew that my psychosomatic illness had a very somatic cause, so did my gratitude to Dr. Gerson. How different the face of med-icine might be today had he received in this country the recognition he'd been on the verge of receiving in his own. How different my own fate might have been had I not had a friend whose life his therapy had saved.

I wish I could say that I never lost faith, but I did; that even during the darkest moments I knew I would be healed, but I didn't. Doubt was never farther away than the next flare-up, and each time despair got a hold on my spirit, the only thing that kept me from giving up was—well, giving up.

Often, I felt again like that child who ran to her mother for help when ill, knowing the only help available was prayer. When prayer failed, which it did on occasion, she would call a Christian Science practitioner to give me "absent treatment." No doubt it was fortunate for us both that I was born a healthy and resilient child.

Looking back on those rare but worrying nights, my strongest memory is not of any particular illness, since none was diagnosed at the time, but of a kind of spiritual confusion. Secretly, I feared my faith would not be strong enough were I to face a life-or-death crisis. And if faith should fail, what then? Beyond Christian Science lay a scary world of doctors and hospitals, of mysterious procedures and forbidden arts, and because that world was unknown and its arts forbidden, the thought that I might have to rely on it one day filled me with fear.

Not until I was in my thirties did the crisis occur. Had it not brought me close to death, I doubt that anything could have torn me away from my faith—the one immutable force in my life.

Now, forty years on, and with the only person I could turn to a continent away, I'd begun to wonder if long-distance healing had been woven into the pattern of my life.

In December the black dog of depression returned, dragging me deeper into a dark and desolate place. I should have known that depression was part of the cleansing process, for pesticides poison the brain as well as the body, but reason vanishes when a voice inside one's head keeps saying, *What is the use? What is it all for?*

Lurching from flare-up to flare-up, from flu-like fevers to chronic fatigue to aches of bewildering origin, I asked the question every sufferer has asked since the dawn of time: *Why me? Why this?* When I thought of the years that stretched before me, my discouragement grew, for I knew it would take more than eighteen months to purge my body of its poisons. Why shouldn't it take years to get rid of what it had taken half a lifetime to acquire?

There were nights when self-pity scratched at the soul and I longed for the touch of a human hand in the dark—consoling myself with the thought that at least I wasn't burdening a husband or lover with the therapy's off-putting demands.

How much of what kept me going was trust in the process and how much sheer doggedness, I cannot say. Part of what sustained me when days were darkest was the thought that others might be going through a similar trial. If the therapy worked for me, then it might work for them.

By mid-December, I had become semi-deranged—yearning for flare-ups one moment as proofs of progress—then fearing they were proofs of defeat when they came. And defeat seemed imminent the day I rang Charlotte with a litany of despair.

"…And even my grip on reality seems to be weakening, Charlotte," I concluded.

"But that's *fine!*" she exclaimed. "You're right on schedule, having completed your fourth month. How often are you taking the castor oil? Only once a week? Make it twice for a while."

Ah well, what doesn't kill me makes me stronger. Or sicker.

One day, when releasing an enema, I passed what appeared to be a long piece of string. Wondering how such an object could have entered my body, on closer inspection I realized it must be a worm. The poor thing must have come to a nasty end during one of my flare-ups, I concluded, for given the rich nutritional environment I was providing, no sensible worm would have wanted to leave. Hoping to preserve it, I seized a nearby comb and tried to retrieve it from the bowl, but it kept sliding off the plastic handle, so I abandoned the effort.

As the months dragged by, I began to chafe at the social restrictions the therapy imposed. Friends could visit and I could visit them, taking my juice in a thermos, but the carefree pleasures I had once taken for granted were now a thing of the past. Gone were weekend seminars in the country, cozy dinners in ethnic restaurants, attending a play, ignoring the hour. Would I ever again know moments of sheer light-hearted fun?

Bored with my world's diminishing horizons, I decided one evening to throw Gerson to the winds, as it were, and have some friends in for dinner. Surely, I deserved one night of self-indulgence after all these months of self-denial.

"Guess what, Isilda?" I announced, cornering her in the kitchen. "We're going to have a dinner party! What do you think of that?"

She glanced up from the chopping board with a scowl.

"What? You make your friends eat this food-with-no-taste?"

"Of course not," I laughed, pinching a leaf of romaine to chew on while having a think. "It will be a proper meal, with wine and cheese and … let's see, perhaps a ratatouille."

"A what?"

"It's a vegetable dish. Don't worry, I'll help you make it. Of course, not all the vegetables can be organic, but it shouldn't matter just this once."

"You no give your friends this juices," she warned, beheading a carrot with a vigorous chop. "I no make extra juices!"

"I wouldn't dream of it," I assured her.

In the event, the dinner was delicious, the company convivial, and the headache I woke up with the next morning a beaut. *It's not fair!* I wailed to an indifferent God. *I didn't even touch the wine!*

Around this time, it occurred to me that I hadn't craved a potato chip or a piece of chocolate since the therapy began. But then, where would such cravings find room in a stomach awash with juice? Of course, had someone placed a bowl of chips before me and left the room, I could not have vouched for my self-restraint, but the addictive element—that craving at odd hours of the day or night—was gone. This seemed as remarkable to me as Beata's release from a thirty-year nicotine addiction or the shrinking of a tumor. Dared I hope that my days of cowering before telluric forces might also be numbered?

I was anticipating this happy prospect when two friends came to dinner on Christmas Eve and again I abandoned my diet. Had the ensuing distress been merely pain I could have taken a pill, but there were no drugs for this kind of internal anarchy—no escape from the chaos of drugs themselves. What can you do when you feel you are losing your mind? Where can you go when you want to jump out of your skin?

It took more faith than I could muster that night to believe that I would be any nearer recovery by the end of 1986. I wandered to the window and stared out at the sky. The night was without a star. Where, I wondered, in that clouded heaven was the star to guide me? Where the King of Peace? Hiding, both of them—like that sage on the mountaintop.

No star. No guide. No peace. Only endless, unremitting night.

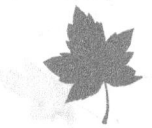

CHAPTER TWENTY-SEVEN

In January '86, I came upon a book about the changes in animal behavior before an earthquake. Quakes being of singular interest to Californians, I was curious to know more about the subject. The book was titled *When the Snakes Awake,* and its author, Helmut Tributsch, had culled reports from around the world of the anomalous behavior of animals hours or even days before an earthquake.

Noting how well-water changes before a quake, becoming cloudy or discolored, Tributsch concludes that some sort of geophysical process takes place in the ground, which acts as a forewarning to sensitive animals—and to sensitive people as well:

> During a severe earthquake, the sensations of sensitive people escalate greatly.... Certain people whose health has been undermined by illness or addiction seem to be extraordinarily sensitive to an approaching earthquake.

People whose health has been undermined by illness....

In a section titled "Human Earthquake Premonition," an Italian scientist in the province of Piedmont described the physiological reactions that were experienced by certain people prior to an earthquake in 1808:

> The more nervous people were seized, for some time before the tremors, by a certain inexplicable restlessness, by a kind of trembling and pounding of the heart.

On reading this description, I felt a sudden click of remembrance. That last night at the clinic … my pounding heart … the mounting anxiety …could they have been premonitory symptoms of the quake that was to rock Mexico City thirty-eight hours later? The very idea seemed absurd, yet the experience of a writer who lived through a severe earthquake in Copiapo, Chile, in 1822, sounded eerily familiar. Describing the disaster signal as "an inexplicable condition of the nervous system that manifests itself before any other sign," he continued:

> Before we hear the sound, or at least are fully conscious of hearing it, we are made sensible, I do not know how, that something uncommon is going to happen; everything seems to change color; our thoughts are chained immovably down; the whole world appears to be in disorder; all nature looks different to what it is wont to do; and we feel quite subdued and overwhelmed by some invisible power, beyond human control or apprehension.

This passage described so vividly the disordered energies revealed by my rod and color wheel that night, that I read on avidly.

According to Tributsch, the average span of time between an observed behavior anomaly and an earthquake can be anywhere from two hours to two days, although he doesn't indicate how near to the epicenter one must be. The quake in Mexico City registered 8.1 on the Richter scale, but the clinic was almost 1,500 miles away.

As for the strange revival of my hair the next morning—if one considers hair to be analogous to a growing plant, then that phenomenon, too, might have been a harbinger of the quake to come. Tributsch cites examples of flowers, trees, and shrubs blooming out of season weeks before an earthquake.

Referring to these anomalies, he comments:

> These types of examples do not seem too numerous, and very few people mention them.… It may be that in the rest of the world similar phenomena are simply not acknowledged because the observers lack sophistication and because the catastrophe does not happen.

If I hadn't chanced upon his book, it wouldn't have occurred to me to link my body's behavior that night with the upheaval that was to strike Mexico a day and a half later. And if it hadn't been for my modest dowsing knowledge, I wouldn't have known that the cause of my physical distress was a massive change in the environment. But why did my symptoms lessen the next day as we drove to the airport? Was it because the car was moving away from the quake's epicenter?

Intriguing though these speculations were, without some means of proving them, they would remain mere conjecture, since I was unlikely to be in the same situation again. I recorded these thoughts in my diary and would have forgotten them, had it not been for my visit home that December, which happened to coincide with what I can only describe as a timely gift from Mother Nature.

The New Year in London began much as the old with morning headaches, waves of sickness, and hair that clung to my scalp like fur on a wet dog's back. Why linger longer on this planet, I wondered, when so much of what I cherish is being polluted or destroyed?

Isilda, too, was growing more disobliging by the day, her small dark eyes narrowing more often, her hands crossing more defiantly over her apron to denote disapproval. Silent and sullen, she marched ahead of me on the way to the greengrocer, asserting her dominance by the distance she put between us.

No week went by without her grumbling about the juices, and lately she'd been getting the sequence wrong—like an actor stuck in a long-running play who grows bored and begins to forget his lines.

Isilda, however, could leave in September—or tomorrow, as she kept reminding me, whereas I was stuck with an indefinite run.

Quite simply, Isilda needed a change. And so did I.

In the seventh month of the therapy that feeling of a mini-generator running under my skin returned. Alarmed at this seeming setback, I rang Charlotte.

"Based on what you're telling me about your symptoms," she said, "you may be detoxifying too fast. I suggest you reduce the juices to six." (Isilda *will* be pleased, I thought.) "But don't be too tied down to the intensive therapy," she warned. "Do what your body tells you to do."

"But my body keeps telling me it hasn't a clue, Charlotte."

She left a pause. "Have you taken much Valium in the past?" she asked.

"I was taking two a day before my divorce, with two sleeping pills at night, but the only Valium I've had since is the tranquilizer they give you before an operation, which I don't need."

"Tranquilizers are much harder to get rid of than chemicals," said Charlotte. "Psychotropic drugs stay in the body for years, but doctors never diagnose Valium poisoning because it can't be detected. Anyway, few of them believe it exists. The benzodiazepines and antidepressants will cause burning and hot flushes and hair loss."

Then that fire in the rectum, my flushes and thinning hair ... could they have been caused by tranquillizers I hadn't taken for years?

Isilda reduced the juices accordingly, but it was the end of April before I was able to sleep comfortably in my bed. By then, there were even days when I felt quite well. It was this paradox of feeling fine one moment and ghastly the next that made environmental illness so hard for doctors to diagnose, and so easy for the unknowing to dismiss.

On April 28, a nuclear reactor at Chernobyl, in the Soviet Union, raged out of control. The first radioactive clouds reached England on the first of May, accompanied by official assurances that "The levels are too low to present any danger." How did they know? By the time the full danger is known, there may be no one left to lie to.

In the forty-second week of the therapy, I had a severe migraine attack that made me glad Isilda was off that day, so I could suffer in peace. As the date for her departure drew near, her bullying increased. Each Iberian oath issuing from the kitchen, each "you-no-like-I-go" ultimatum, made me yearn for a placid, monosyllabic Swede as her replacement in September.

I was at my lowest ebb in June when an incident occurred involving my daughter Amy that plunged me into a state of impotent despair. Unable to protect her, I fell into a mindless fury. The anger flare-up had been long in coming, but when it came, the rage I had suppressed for a lifetime exploded with a frenzy I was powerless to contain. I grabbed a large cushion and began to pummel it with my fists, hurling blows on everything and everyone I blamed for turning me into a wimp—and for good measure I beat the hell out of that scorpion self that kept stinging me with its tail. When I tried to sleep, my impotence kept me awake, and when I woke it was still there, pounding away like a fever in my skull. I wanted to weep, curse, howl, shake my fist at heaven, strike out at *everything* that was turning my world upside down, and all I could do was beat the stuffing out of an innocent pillow!

Even in my unhinged state I remembered how certain I was that *I* would not be subject to the same angry flare-ups Beata had experienced. Yet here I was, stomping all over her well-trodden footsteps, like a beastly child—behaving as badly as she did, and being ashamed of myself into the bargain.

For days I functioned on the periphery of amnesia, forgetting appointments, losing the thread of a thought in mid-sentence, and losing my short-term memory altogether. Like an unmanned train hurtling toward disaster, I was manifesting all the signs of toxic psychosis.

Tooling along Brompton Road in the wrong direction one day, I mistook the row of cars facing me for being parked, instead of a line of traffic waiting for the light to change. When I realized my mistake, I seem to have been jolted out of a trance. I made a quick U-turn and, as the cars moved forward, squeezed into the queue—right in front of a police car, which promptly flashed its lights for me to pull over.

Cringing with shame, I watched in the side-view mirror as a young officer got out of his car, walked up to mine, and bent down to address me through my open window:

"Are you aware, madam," he said, with pained courtesy, "that you were in the lane for oncoming cars and were therefore creating a traffic hazard?"

"I know ... I mean, no I didn't realize," I stammered. "I'm sorry, officer, but you see, I've been ill and I'm afraid I haven't been thinking clearly."

"Do you think you should be driving in this condition?" he asked, not unkindly.

"I don't think I should be *living* in this condition," I said.

The officer must have had a soft heart, for he let me off with just a warning. All the same, I was so alarmed by the incident, that I rang Charlotte when I got home.

"A *very* good sign!" she exclaimed. "Normally, anger and confusion don't surface until the main part of the healing is over. In most cases, the chemicals in the brain are the last to mobilize into the bloodstream."

Tell that to the policeman! I thought, and to anyone else I had alienated while the balance of my mind was disturbed. By July, however, the brain fog subsided and I felt reasonably normal again.

With Isilda's departure in September drawing near, I began to look for her replacement in August.

"I think I've found someone, Isilda," I said. "She's a Polish lady—late thirties I think, and seems quite pleasant. Her name is Bronya. I've invited her to come by tomorrow and watch you make a juice, so that she'll be familiar with the procedure when she begins."

"Why you invite?" demanded Isilda, angrily. "I no like she watch me when I work."

"Come, now, Isilda, it's only for an hour."

As I might have foreseen, Isilda was so curt with the young woman, making no effort to be helpful or even civil, that I had to apologize to Bronya when saying goodbye to her at the door.

"Really, Isilda," I said, returning to the kitchen, "you might at least have *tried* to be polite." But she affected not to hear. Turning away, she grabbed a dish cloth and made a pointed show of cleaning the juicing machine.

Two weeks before she was to leave, Isilda came into the sitting room one evening lugging the suitcase she was going to send on ahead to Portugal.

"I bring for you to look inside before I send," she said. "See I no steal nothing."

"Steal?" I echoed, surprised. "When have I ever questioned your honesty, Isilda? Of course I won't look through your things."

Turning away, she trundled the suitcase back to her room. Days later, after running an errand for me at the chemist's, she thrust her open palm at me with the change.

"Here, you count, see I do not steal."

"I will *not* count," I snapped. "What *is* all this about stealing, Isilda? When have I ever mistrusted you!"

As though trust was an added affront, her mouth tightened and she marched off to the kitchen, leaving me to wonder if I could endure fourteen more days of Isilda without closing my hands around her throat.

The night before her departure, she confronted me after dinner.

"How much money you give me when I go?" she asked, her gimlet eyes narrowing. "Four-week vacation, yes?"

Even after a year, Isilda's audacity could still astonish me. I had no legal obligation to give her a penny, but four weeks was what I had planned. Being *ordered* to do so, however, was the last straw. Anger loosened my reluctant tongue, and I lost my temper.

"What makes you think I *wouldn't* do the right thing by you, Isilda?" I demanded. "Have I ever cheated you? Tell me, have I? Frankly, your attitude these past months has driven me up the wall, and as for your complaints, I've had *those* right up to here! At times your behavior has been so … so *uncalled* for, it was all I could do to keep from telling you off!"

Stunned by this outburst, which took us both by surprise, Isilda was speechless. If only *I* had been as well, for even as the words left my lips I regretted them.

"Oh, I'm sorry, Isilda," I said, my anger collapsing like a dud soufflé. "Forgive me, I've been under a strain lately … a personal matter and … well, it's just that you *could* have been more helpful at times. Please forgive me."

But Isilda, for whom a grievance was like gold, was not about to forgive. Turning on her heel she swept wordlessly away, closing her bedroom door with an eloquent bang. Sick with remorse, I spent the rest of the evening reproaching myself for my loss of control.

Determined to patch things up before she left, the next morning I waited until Isilda had brought her bags into the hall before trying to slip the vacation money into her coat pocket, but she pushed my hand angrily away. Seizing her bags, she walked to the door, pausing only long enough to deliver a parting shot:

"I think now, when I go, you fumigate my room, yes?"

As I watched her dark figure disappear down the stairs, I wondered if any part of my life made sense anymore. Was there something in me that brought out the madness in others, or was I even madder than I could bring myself to believe? With a leaden heart I closed the door, telling myself these things were sent to try us. No doubt Isilda had found *me* as hard to live with as I had found her—although, in a funny way, I was going to miss her. She may have been difficult, but she was never dull.

When I think of her now, I see her sitting in a Portuguese piazza, enjoying her *Bacalhau* and Madeira, while regaling friends with tales of "all this juices" she had to make for a crazy American who was so crackers she kept putting coffee up her behind.

Ah, well, with luck, Isilda will never have to know that it worked.

INVISIBLE ENEMY

CHAPTER TWENTY-EIGHT

Bronya had been in situ less than a week when I began to suspect that I had exchanged one domestic problem for another. There had been no hint at our meeting of the manic carnivore who would fill the flat with the fumes of frying meat, while making heavy weather of the simplest task. Slow and disorganized, she fussed over trifles while leaving important things undone, such as reorganizing the cutlery drawer while leafy vegetables wilted on the draining board. Juices arrived erratically, and dishes piled up in the sink until after dinner. Since she rarely ate before nine, the chaos in the kitchen was chronic.

Too disheartened to look for someone else, I told myself not to be such a bloody perfectionist and tried to avert my eyes. Aspects of her behavior, however, made me suspect that at some time in the past Bronya might have suffered a nervous breakdown. Disarmed at first by the gentleness of her voice and manner, I soon discovered they cloaked a nature every bit as controlling as Isilda's. Four weeks into the job, she demanded an increase in the salary she had described as "generous" the day she was engaged.

At first, I attributed her mood swings to the premenstrual tension she had warned me about, but there was no cyclical pattern to her compulsive-addictive behavior. If I entered the kitchen after dinner, I found her standing there with a dreamy look in her eyes, lovingly polishing a saucepan that already gleamed like a burnished jewel. She refused to use the washing machine, even though we did our laundry separately, "because," she explained, "you sometimes put your underpants in the same load with the sheets!"

Unable to feel much guilt about this, I dismissed her concern as just another eccentricity. One day, however, after she had removed my laundry from the dryer, she approached my desk holding something aloft between her forefinger and thumb with an air of fastidious distaste.

"Look!" she cried, "*Look* what I found in your laundry! A pubic hair!"

I sighed. "Well, at least it's a clean pubic hair," I observed, and went on with my work.

Although Bronya's need to control was subtler than Isilda's, it was not long before my inner wimp was caving in to her demands. What was it in me that brought out the bully in women? Did I really need another dominatrix in my life?

In the course of my reading that fall, I came upon a reference to the HealthMed Detoxification Program in Los Angeles. A three- to four-week course based on dry saunas and aerobic exercise, it was conceived by the late L. Ron Hubbard of Scientology fame, presumably to detoxify those of his followers who were hooked on drugs. It had also been shown, however, to help victims of environmental illness.

Like most Gerson patients, I had wished there could be an easier, less labor-intensive method of detoxifying the body, but I doubted a month of saunas could achieve the same results. I was also leery of the Hubbard connection.

When I lived in Paris in the 1960s, an acquaintance invited me to attend a Scientology meeting and gave me a copy of Hubbard's book, *Dianetics,* to read. As I had recently left the church I was open to new ideas, but I found aspects of the movement dubious, and Hubbard's book unfinishable. I was not surprised to learn that in a previous incarnation he had been a writer of science fiction. Was HealthMed a front for luring the addicted into the religion, I wondered, or was it a valid program for detoxifying the body?

Although I was now well on the way to recovery and able to live comfortably in my flat, the problems that had driven me from it before were still there. I was therefore prepared to try anything that might hasten the healing process. I rang the clinic in Los Angeles and spoke with the director, Michael Wisner. After explaining my problem, I asked:

"Do you think saunas could rid my body of its remaining chemicals—even of heavy metals?"

"Well, the program was tested on some people in Michigan who were exposed to PBDEs in 1973," he said. "Because of a mistake at the Michigan Chemical Corporation, massive amounts of flame retardant got mixed into cattle feed. Not only did the livestock have to be destroyed, but people were eating the contaminated meat and dairy products for nine months *before* the cause of the widespread illness was discovered. This left close to nine million people with PBDEs in their tissues and blood.

"During a twenty-day sauna program," Wisner continued, "twenty-five percent of the toxins were removed, with corresponding improvement in reaction times and long-term memory."

A promising result, to be sure, but that still left seventy-five percent of toxins in the system, and one couldn't take saunas forever. Even after fourteen months on the therapy, I was still shedding poisons that must have been in my body fat for years.

Wisner confirmed that Dr. Rae was building a sauna modeled on the one in L.A., and I told him about my test for chlorinated pesticides.

"I know the test," he said, "but it only measures the chemicals in the blood; it's the toxins in the body fat that matter." I agreed. "Before the program begins," he added, "we do tests to determine your levels."

Since I was going to be in Beverly Hills at Christmas, visiting my family, I decided to do the program while there, as it might prove a useful adjunct to the therapy.

Reflecting on the way coming events cast their shadow before them, it occurred to me that food must have been part of my destiny from the day I was born.

My adoptive father was a restaurateur whose catering career began during the Great Depression. Although he was a good man and a caring father, he had an ungovernable temper that was a frequent cause of distress when I was young. Most of his outbursts took place at the dinner table—as did our many clashes over politics, when I grew older. And now here I was, as dependent on food for the sake of survival as my father had been for the sake of earning a living. I saw once more his wholesale supplier delivering those two-inch steaks to our home, shuddered anew at the memory of that knife-sharpening ritual that preceded his dismemberment of the Sunday roast, and yearned again (though less longingly now) for those rich desserts that had crowned our Lucullan meals.

What would my father have said then, I wondered, had he known that forty years on, my health—perhaps even my life—would depend on a diet the very opposite of the one he was providing at home?

Looking back, I felt I had been twice saved: First, by adoption into a loving home filled with self-indulgence, and now, by a discipline of the most stringent self-denial—only this time, one that I myself had chosen to adopt.

CHAPTER TWENTY-NINE

My Christmas-at-a-clinic for 1986 was spent in a sauna, sweating out the old year and sweating in the new. The flight from London had been as pleasant as any trip can be when confined in a metal box for nine hours sharing germs with two hundred other people.

Michael Wisner had booked me into a motor hotel on Beverly Boulevard, chosen for its proximity to the clinic and for its freedom from the sort of chemical products I'd have been exposed to in a modern, well-maintained hotel. The motel's maintenance was minimal, but at least there was an excellent health food store two blocks away.

I checked into HealthMed on December 15 for the usual preliminary tests, to which were added toxicology screens and a hair analysis for heavy metals. When I told the doctor I was doing the Gerson Therapy, she asked me to suspend the coffee enemas while I was there. I said I would try.

Two days later, the program began. I was given a controlled dose of niacin (vitamin B_3) to trigger the release of toxins into the bloodstream before doing a twenty-minute obligatory jog around the block (for the less fit, a brisk walk).

"The jog acts with the niacin to increase the depth of circulation into your tissues," explained the supervisor, a beetle-browed fellow named Faxon, who took our blood pressure each morning and whose droll, laconic manner masked an ever-vigilant eye. "You must jog or walk in pairs and never sauna alone," he warned, "because you could have a flashback while unattended." The flashback was the HealthMed version of the Gerson flare-up.

My jogging partners that morning were Sam—a balding appliance salesman in his sixties from Bakersfield—and Doris, a retired school-teacher from Georgia, who was also staying at the motel. We agreed to walk briskly instead of jog, so that we could exchange our case histories along the way.

"I've been a heavy smoker since my teens," said Sam, "and I like to tinker in the garage on weekends—you know, make things like furniture and stuff. I thought I was a pretty healthy guy until a few years ago, when I developed emphysema and started having a lot of other physical problems."

Doris's story was similar to that of Louise, my housemate at Willie Mae's.

"One of the cleaners at school dumped a gallon of chlorine into the sink of the utility room next to my classroom," she said. "I had barely recovered from that when, without my realizing it, the pilot light on my gas stove went out and I was exposed to carbon monoxide. A friend who worked in the office at school told me she got sick from the acetone that outgassed from the copier she used every day."

By the time I had skipped through my own story, our aerobic walk was over, and we changed into our swimsuits (nudity was forbidden in the mixed sauna). Faxon recorded our starting weight and gave us each a clipboard, a form sheet, a pencil, and two paper cups containing salt and potassium tablets.

"You're to record the time each session begins and ends," he instructed, "along with the number of salt and potassium tablets you take, the glasses of water you drink, any symptoms that occur, and the total amount of sauna time completed each day. Heat exposure is from ten to thirty minutes, no more, followed by a ten- to fifteen-minute cooling-down period, with a cold shower and rest between each sauna. This is very important," he said.

"The sauna room is ventilated and kept at about 140 degrees, not the usual 200 degrees maintained in health clubs. The lower temperature increases the excretion of toxins through the sweating mechanism without placing a strain on the heart. You'll be given daily supplements to replace the electrolytes, minerals, and vitamins lost during the sweating, with emphasis on calcium and magnesium, which you'll take as a drink."

The goal was five hours of sauna time per day, taken in half-hour segments. Faxon advised me to limit my first session to twenty minutes, which I would have done anyway, since by then I was feeling slightly ill. When I went to the rest area, he gave me a glass of the calcium-magnesium drink (Cal-Mag), which I quite liked.

During the second session, a strange odor emerged from my armpits. This was disconcerting, as I had never had a body odor problem. I expressed my concern to Doris, who was in her second week of the program.

"Don't worry," she said. "There was a girl here last week who gave off a strong body odor for two days. It must be the toxins coming out through your pores."

Later, when I queried Faxon about this, he confirmed that it was a common occurrence. "It's one of the detox signs we see in people who have taken street drugs," he said.

"But I've never taken street drugs."

"Well, it can also happen if you've had a lot of medicinal drugs—old antibiotics, anesthetics, tranquilizers, sleeping pills, painkillers—that sort of thing."

Why, then, I wondered, hadn't this occurred on the therapy? Did saunas reach parts of the body the juices missed? More symptoms emerged, and by the end of the third session, Faxon decided I'd had enough for the first day. He weighed me again and gave me a large drink of unsaturated oils mixed with kefir.

"The drink enhances fatty oil exchange and promotes fecal evacuation," he explained. "Only forty percent of toxins can be eliminated through the sweat glands."

In that case, I thought, why forbid enemas while provoking diarrhea?

On the walk back to the motel I felt thoroughly whacked. My head ached, my neck hurt, my right ear kept popping, and my left hip had developed an arthritic twinge.

Altogether, a promising first day.

On the nineteenth, I woke at half past five, feeling as though I had the flu. The symptom cleared during the first sauna but returned after the break, with more nausea and more body odor leaving my pores.

I had discovered that all the employees were Scientologists, although distinctly reticent about discussing the fact. No Hubbard books were on display, nor were there any pictures of Cap'n Ron looking jaunty in his yachting cap.

"The clinic's purpose is solely therapeutic," Faxon assured me, when I asked him about their absence. "It has nothing to do with drawing people into the religion." I saw no reason to doubt his statement during my four weeks at HealthMed.

Two young women appeared in the sauna that morning—former patients who were having one of the free maintenance sessions available to those who have completed the program. Bright and chatty, they described some of the symptoms they had witnessed in the sauna.

"When I was here a year ago," said the one with brown hair and dark, intelligent eyes, "there was a middle-aged guy who'd been a heavy smoker. His legs started to ooze a brown liquid, as though nicotine was coming out of his pores. And I heard there was an LSD user who began tripping so badly they made him stay in the sauna until he'd sweated it all out."

"What happened to me," said her bikini-clad friend, blonde hair pulled back in a ponytail, "was that my nose became all swollen and painful, and blue circles appeared under my eyes. I'd had a nose job two years before—and not only that, my body gave off an odor that smelled funny, like sodium pentothal, which is the anesthetic they told me I was given at the time of my op."

I recalled Charlotte's story about the patient with the suture that had worked its way out of her nose years after a rhinoplasty. Which chemicals were working their way out of my armpits? I wondered. Chlorine? Dieldrin? Hexachlorobenzene?

Sam, bless his heart, was a bit of a drone, humming "Danny Boy" in the sauna and describing his symptoms in Proustian detail to anyone who would listen. Seeking a quieter ambience, I decided to try the smaller sauna on the floor below, which Faxon had told us we were not to use if alone. I opened the door to find a young bloke there listening to a ball game on a transistor radio. Changing my mind, I returned to the sauna upstairs. Better the drone I knew....

On the twenty-first, I learned that a patient of Dr. Rae's had arrived from Texas. She appeared in the sauna the following day—a beautiful young woman, Lynn, whose slightly slurred speech and unsteady movements suggested she'd been exposed to a severe chemical assault.

Halfway through the first session she rose and made her way out of the sauna. I assumed she had gone home, but when I went into the rest area for my break, I found her there, drinking a glass of Cal-Mag. Curious to know her story, I introduced myself as a former patient of Dr. Rae and asked if she would mind telling me what had brought her to HealthMed.

"My husband and I built our million-dollar dream home in Dallas," she began, "but somehow the builder made a mistake. A pipe carrying trichloroethylene—that's a chemical used in dry cleaning— was installed the wrong way, so that it emptied through a drain into my dressing room. My dressing room also happened to be the office for my decorating business. I spent hours there each day, inhaling the chemical without realizing it, and it attacked my nervous system.

"We're suing the builder, of course," she added, "but our finances are running low. Meanwhile, my husband is also ill, and because the house is too contaminated to live in, our three young children are staying in a hotel with a helper."

My first thought was that Lynn should not be doing the program, she was much too ill.

"I hope you're not here alone," I said.

"My husband couldn't afford to come," she explained, "so I'm staying in a motel."

On establishing that it was the same one as mine, I invited her to join Doris and me when we walked to the clinic in the morning.

"Thank you," she said, "but I come later, because I can't jog or do the fast walk."

"Oh, of course. Well, then, perhaps on the walk back?"

Faxon arrived to check on Lynn, and wisely decided to send her back to the motel to rest. I returned to the sauna and told Doris about our conversation.

"I'm concerned about Lynn walking alone to the clinic, Doris. Frankly, I'm not sure she should be here at all."

"Maybe we could give her our room numbers in case she has an emergency during the night," said Doris—"although," she added, "I don't know what we could do for her if she did."

Neither did I. Later that day, I confided my concern to the director.

"What worries me, Michael, is that someone as ill as Lynn—especially if the chemicals in her body are released too quickly into her bloodstream—could end up in a worse state than when she arrived. That's what happened to me when I left the ECU."

"Don't worry," he said, "we're keeping a close eye on her. In fact, we've scheduled some extra tests to decide if she should stay in the program."

Walking to the motel with Doris that afternoon, I saw her pass her hand over her forehead several times.

"Are you all right, Doris?" I asked.

"It must be the perfume that girl had on in the changing room," she said. "It's brought back the headache I'd gotten rid of in the sauna."

"I know, it bothered me, too. I'm surprised they don't have a sign somewhere forbidding the use of scented products in the changing areas as well as the saunas."

"I don't know how we can detoxify if we keep being exposed to the chemicals that made us sick in the first place," grumbled Doris.

It was the litany of our lives, the lament of chemical victims every-where as we topple from our perches, our toxic bodies warning of the dangers that lie ahead. My heart ached for Doris, since I knew she would need more than saunas to repair the damage caused by that careless ac-cident at school. I had told her about the Gerson Therapy, but she said she couldn't afford it.

"I wonder why we're so heedless about our health, Doris," I mused—"I mean, as a nation, and so indifferent to the environmental problems we're creating for generations to come."

"Well, if we keep procreating the way we're doing," she said, "there won't be any environment left for future generations to worry about."

"Of course, that's the bottom line, isn't it: the population explo-sion—the problem no politician will touch for fear of treading on cultural or religious toes." [2]

"At least the Chinese have tried to deal with the problem by limit-ing families to one child," said Doris.

"Yes, but what if an only child dies? And what about the women in Africa, who have no control over their fertility? One has only to see a picture of a starving child to know that Oedipus was right. 'Not to be born is best!' "

"Instead," said Doris, "we keep breeding and polluting, as though the planet's resources are inexhaustible."

"It's not even as though we need all the things that are creating the toxic waste being dumped into landfills."

"No, but replacing them with organic materials would be prohib-itively expensive."

"No more so than the cost of cleaning up after an oil spill. No more than the cost of our declining health and soaring medical bills. But who in Washington will defy the chemical lobbies, with their deep pockets and welcome bribes?"

"Well, let's hope that *someone* in government wakes up before it's too late," sighed Doris, without conviction.

2 David Attenborough, the famous naturalist, observed: "There are three times as many people on earth as when I started making natural history programs 60 years ago.... It seems to me there is a huge moral responsibility we have towards this planet." *The London Sunday Times,* September, 2008.

"Even if someone wakes up tomorrow," I said, "it's already too late."
As long ago as 1984, Lee N. Davis wrote in *The Corporate Alchemists*:

> Each year we are letting loose small quantities of new
> materials that do not occur naturally. Many have been
> specifically designed to be potent and toxic. Others become
> dangerous when overused, misused, or mixed with other
> substances. Such chemicals, borne by wind and water, have
> worked their way to the remotest portions of the globe
> and the farthest reaches of the atmosphere. We are literally
> surrounded by poisons. Their number increases annually. We
> have no idea what their ultimate effects will be.

Except that now, in the year 2016, we do.

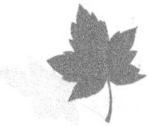

CHAPTER THIRTY

On the twenty-second, I woke feeling headachy and vaguely ill. I was also inexpressibly tired, so I assumed I was having a flashback. Although I had been asked to eschew coffee enemas while there, I needed to get the toxins out of my bloodstream as quickly as possible. Without their swift elimination, I'm not sure I would have stayed in the program. I did feel guilty about breaking one of the rules—though not so guilty I didn't break another one that day, when Sam broke into song and I fled again to the sauna below, this time happily unoccupied.

We were joined in the changing room that morning by a pretty young college student, Jennifer, whose auburn curls fell in ringlets around her cheeks. Fresh-faced and chubby, she looked much too wholesome to be the drug-taking type—so, in my nosy way, I asked her what had brought her to HealthMed.

"I'm here to get NutraSweet® out of my system," she said.

"NutraSweet?"

"Yes, that's aspartame. It's in all the diet colas. I've been trying to lose weight and was drinking lots of colas at college because I thought they were safe, but on the last day of school I passed out in my room. I don't know how long I was unconscious. When I came to, almost everyone had gone and I couldn't move. I was paralyzed. Fortunately, someone found me in time and the paralysis was only temporary, but it has affected my mind. By the time my doctor identified NutraSweet as the cause, some of the cells in my brain had been destroyed."

"But what makes him suspect aspartame?" I asked, more likely candidates springing to mind.

"Because the tests confirmed it," said Jennifer. "It's in all the sweeteners. We found out that when aspartame is subjected to temperatures over 80 degrees it breaks down into methanol, and methanol breaks down and converts to formaldehyde, even in body heat."

"But if that's so, it should have been withdrawn years ago. Has your doctor reported this to the FDA?"

"Oh, yes, he has, but he doesn't think they'll do anything about it. He says the FDA protects the food and drug industries, not the public. Besides, Monsanto, which makes aspartame, funds the American Diabetes Association, so the ADA puts pressure on the FDA not to remove it. It's all about money."

All about money, when it should be all about health.

The problems with aspartame have been known to the FDA for years, yet they let Monsanto incorporate it into 6,000 food products, such as diet sodas, sugar-free desserts, candy, yogurts, chewing gum, and those packets of sugar substitutes, such as Equal®, that sit so deceitfully on restaurant tables. Jennifer's story was not the first to reveal the duplicity of government bureaucracies that were formed to protect the public but in practice protect the drug companies instead.

In her book *The Secret History of the War on Cancer,* Devra Davis cites a 1969 study of aspartame that was done with seven infant monkeys. "After a year of drinking milk flavored with the stuff," she writes, "one was dead and five had suffered severe epileptic seizures." A later study showed that "aspartame paired with the food flavoring monosodium glutamate produced brain tumors in rats." Manufacturers now hide MSG under a dozen different names, such as "hydrolyzed soy protein," etc. It is in far more foods than consumers are aware of—or than our government allows us to know.

On the twenty-seventh, the soles of my feet began to ache in the sauna and a strong odor issued again from my pores. Lynn, however, showed a marked improvement that day. Her speech was fluent and her balance had greatly improved. It was the first time she had stayed for the last sauna, so Doris and I invited her to walk back with us to the motel.

To avoid the traffic fumes on Beverly Boulevard, we went through a back alley that led past a row of garages behind the apartment buildings. One of the garage doors ahead was open, and as we approached it Lynn's legs suddenly buckled and she gasped, "Oh, no!" We caught her in time, catching the whiff of motor oil ourselves, but all the progress Lynn had made in the sauna that day was undone. Somehow we managed to get her to her room, where she collapsed onto the bed.

"Is there anything we can do for you, Lynn?" I asked, knowing there wasn't, as she lay there in distress.

"I need to eat some greens," she whispered, "but I don't have any. Anyway, I don't think I have the strength to fix dinner."

"You don't have to," I said. "I was going to make a salad for dinner, so I'll make enough for two."

Doris stayed with Lynn, while I went downstairs and threw some greens together with a tomato, a hard-boiled egg, some cucumber slices, and a yogurt and chive dressing. After adding some fruit to the tray, I returned to Lynn's room and placed the tray on her nightstand, while Doris helped her into a sitting position.

"I'll be going to the health food store tomorrow, Lynn," I said. "If there's anything you need, I can get it for you."

I made a note of the few items she requested and then, there being nothing more we could do, Doris and I returned to our rooms.

I had lost my appetite and was feeling unwell, so I went to bed. However, I couldn't sleep. Thoughts of Lynn troubled my mind. What further damage had that motor oil exposure done to her fragile immune system? How could a glass of kefir and oils remove enough of the volatile toxins from her overstressed body? Had I chosen saunas as a first resort instead of Gerson, I might have ended up in the same condition as Lynn.

At the health food store the next day, I added flaxseed oil and some bottles of carrot juice to Lynn's list. There couldn't have been a live enzyme left in the juice, but it was better than nothing. When I reached Lynn's room, she was still desperately ill.

"I don't know when I'll be able to do the saunas again," she said, her voice thin with fatigue.

"If I were you I wouldn't try," I said, "not until you've spoken with Michael."

That night I felt restless again and found it hard to sleep. Around 2:00 a.m. I woke feeling as though a small motor was pulsing in my feet. What should I do if an earthquake was imminent, I wondered? Stand in a doorway? Take shelter under a table?

The next morning, I turned on the radio:

> There has been a mild earthquake in the Hayward district of the Bay City area at 7:28 this morning, 3.5 on the Richter scale.

The Hayward district, I learned, was about 300 miles north of Los Angeles—too far, surely, for premonitory vibrations to be felt in Beverly Hills. Still, the distance from Mexico City to La Gloria had been five times greater, although the quake had been five times stronger, too. If my symptoms that night at the clinic had been due, indeed, to the coming temblor, were they weaker this time because the quake was weaker or because my immune system was stronger?

The thought that I might be subject to these forces for the rest of my life was too worrying to contemplate on an empty stomach, so I recorded the quake in my diary and turned my attention to the more tangible matter of food.

Meanwhile, without intending to, I'd been giving Faxon a hard time. I had already blotted my copybook by suggesting that coffee enemas be added to the program. When I told him I had taken one the night before to relieve a headache, he looked aggrieved. When I admitted to one the night before that, he sucked his teeth and scowled. I did feel the teeniest bit guilty about confessing to only two, but, as Heinrich Heine said, "God will forgive me; that's his job."

Doris was ill that day, and Sam, having finished the program, had decamped the day before, so I was assigned a new jogging partner—a lady of a certain age, Mitzi, who was petite, trim, and blondish, with a pixie haircut and personality to match. Her chatter was a welcome change from Sam's lugubrious narratives, and she promised to be an invigorating companion. "I think I should warn you that I'm kind of hyper," she began, as we set out on our power walk. "I mean, I'm so hyper that one of my colleagues at work said to me, 'Mitzi,' she said, 'they could bury you under a concrete slab and you'd come right back up like a weed, even if you had to crack open the concrete!' Tee hee! They all think I'm a card at the office."

Extruding verbiage like ticker tape, Mitzi, who worked in a department store, had the kind of chirpiness that relieves the listener of any obligation to respond. We had gone but a few steps when she cried, "Wait!" I stopped while she reached into the pocket of her gym suit to withdraw a chocolate bar.

"I shouldn't be eating this, you know," she said, unwrapping it with a guilty giggle. "My doctor read me the riot act when I told him I was coming here to get rid of the chemicals in my system. 'Mitzi,' he said, 'I think you're crazy. Your trouble is allergy, *allergy!* And chocolate is the worst thing for you, you've got to give it up!' But I can't," she whimpered, making a moue. "I mean—it's so *addictive!* I would *kill* for chocolate! It's more addictive than sex! Here, want a bite?"

I shook my head. *There but for the grace of Gerson,* thought I. To her credit, Mitzi had a sense of humor about herself, although she did get up the noses of a few people—Faxon's in particular, whose laid-back feathers she kept ruffling by calling him "Fraxon."

"By the way," said Mitzi, as we resumed our walk, "what star sign were you born under?"

"Scorpio. Why?"

"Why, I'm Scorpio, too! How *amazing!* Do you know what your rising sign is?"

"Yes. Cancer."

"I have Gemini rising. No wonder we get on so well. I told Fraxon you're the only person I like to walk with because you walk fast, like me, and are so interesting to talk to. I'm an amateur astrologer, you know, and a very old soul. Oh, it's all there in my chart. You won't believe this, but once, in a former life...."

And so, interminably, on.

That afternoon, I was surprised to see Lynn in the sauna. Her movements, however, suggested someone in the early stages of Alzheimer's. Might that affliction, too, I wondered, have an environmental cause? Faxon wisely sent Lynn back home at the first break. I prayed she would make it back safely to the motel.

Plodding home alone on the last day of the year with low spirits, a raw throat, and a pounding head, I missed Doris's level-headed company. She had finished the program, but was still ill and would be leaving the next day.

That night, I reflected on the absurdity of my situation. Here I was in a run-down motel in my home town on New Year's Eve, when I should have been in London greeting 1987 with a few close friends, a glass of carrot juice, and subdued expectations.

Some time after midnight, I woke with my feet pulsing again in that familiar manner. Though the vibration was weaker this time, it was sufficiently annoying to keep me awake for more than an hour.

The next morning I switched on the radio:

A mild earthquake has occurred in Palm Springs, about 120 miles from Los Angeles, 3.6 on the Richter scale.

CHAPTER THIRTY-ONE

"Oh, yes," said Mitzi, while on our morning walk, "I've been through all that new-age stuff—tarot, channeling, OBEs," (she correctly assumed I would know the acronym for out-of-body experiences). "Once, when I was out of my body, I had the most *amazing* experience! I was traveling in a little spaceship all by myself, faster than the speed of light, when these *amazing* beings appeared! I knew they were cosmic beings, not aliens, because they had no faces and were from a much more advanced civilization. Anyway, while they were showing me my former lives, they took me to the planet Sirius and they said to me, 'Mitzi, you won't remember this, but many lifetimes ago, you were a high priestess here on this planet.'"

"Oh, do tell me—what is Sirius like?"

"Well, it's not like earth at all. The buildings are all round and made of glass and you can walk right through the walls, only of course your feet don't touch the ground. Only very old souls reincarnate on Sirius—those who have lived many lifetimes."

In the sauna, Mitzi was still on her cosmic canter when I thought I felt a slight tremor in the bench. I wanted to ask if she felt it, too, but Mitzi was in full flow, and by the time she drew breath the vibration had ceased. Later that day, a second earthquake was reported near Palm Springs, 3.6 on the Richter scale.

Intrigued by these synchronicities, I looked through the previous entries in my diary to see if a time pattern emerged between the onset of certain symptoms and a quake. Depending on the strength and distance of the temblor, there seemed to be an interval of from four to six hours between the two. I hadn't noted the time of the tremor in the sauna that morning, nor that of the quake that afternoon, but if the former occurred around 10:00 a.m. and the latter between 2:00 and 4:00 p.m., it would have fallen within that range.

All the same, three coincidences did not make a premonition.

That same day, we learned that Lynn had dropped out of the program and was undergoing some neurological tests.

"Her condition has deteriorated rapidly," Faxon told us.

If only we hadn't gone through that alley!

On the fourth, two young women joined us in the sauna.

"We're here to get old LSD out of our systems," one of them told us. "We used to do drugs, but now that we're married and want to have kids, we thought we'd better get clean first."

Listening to their stories, I was grateful—not for the first time—that I had never been tempted by the lure of mind-altering drugs. Also, I was surprised that we hadn't been given any dietary advice with our other instructions. I asked Michael about this later that day.

"We don't believe in imposing an additional burden on people while they're doing the program," he explained.

Burden? Different therapy, different approach: nutrition as burden instead of builder.

The following night I woke in the wee hours with my body humming gently and my feet thrumming as though hooked up to that mini-generator again. The symptoms were stronger this time, so I got up and recorded them in my diary, in case another seismic surprise was on its way.

When I woke later that morning, I turned on the news as usual and learned there had been an earthquake in the Aleutian Islands off Alaska—6.4 on the Richter scale.

Now, it is one thing to sense a disturbance in the earth when the vibrations are under one's feet, so to speak, but when they occur off a distant shore? I had no problem taking the improbable in my stride, thanks to our resident poltergeist in London, but to imagine a connection between a subterranean plate shifting off the coast of Alaska and my central nervous system in Beverly Hills felt like a stretch.

Yet, if the human body can react to an invisible energy line or the noxious emanation from a polluted stream, why shouldn't it sense an impending displacement within the earth itself? After all, earth, sea, and air are all part of one planetary whole, with which we are in constant, if not always conscious, communion.

Still puzzling, however, was why my symptoms were stronger before the more distant quake in the Aleutian Islands than they were before the weaker one in Palm Springs. Tributsch points out that as tsunamis race across the ocean, they pound the rock formations beneath the sea floor, and because sound travels faster through rock than through water, animals sense the vibrations that way and have time to flee.

The means by which humans might also sense the same vibrations was suggested by Giorgio Piccardi, director of the Institute of Physical Chemistry in Florence, Italy, who wrote:

> Water is sensitive to extremely delicate influences and is capable of adapting itself to the most varying circumstances to a degree attained by no other liquid. Perhaps it is even by means of water and the aqueous system that the external forces are able to react on living organisms.

Ever since I could remember, water had been my native element. Much of my childhood was spent at the bottom of a swimming pool, searching for coins my brother and I had thrown in. With scarves attached to my swimsuit, I pretended to be a sinuous undine, tumbling in the silent depths to watch the silken squares make graceful arabesques in my wake. Even my astrological chart was awash with watery signs, including a "grand trine" in water—whatever that meant, though I was sure Mitzi could tell me.

In the sauna that afternoon, Faxon opened the door to tell us that Lynn may have suffered some brain damage and had dropped out of the program.

"Her brother has arrived from Texas to take her home," he added. "She's downstairs now if you want to say goodbye to her."

The shock of seeing Lynn in a wheelchair—so beautiful, and so broken—was heartbreaking. As we each bent down to kiss her good-bye, her eyes filled with tears. I managed to withhold mine until she had gone, but as her brother wheeled her toward the door I slipped a hastily scribbled note into his pocket, urging them to look into the Gerson Therapy. I knew they wouldn't; why should they, when everything else they had tried had failed?

Later, Faxon told us, "Lynn's blood tests showed an exceptionally high level of trichloroethylene in her body—a thousand times higher than it should have been. Trichloroethylene is a dry-cleaning chemical. That's what was coming up through a pipe in her dressing room, which she had been breathing for months."

I was fixing supper on Thursday evening when I thought I felt a faint tremor in my lower legs. I might not have noticed it had it not been for my habit of hypervigilance. For a moment I thought of lying down, since my symptoms were more pronounced when I was prone, but I was hungry, and as the vibration was mild, I decided to eat instead. Later however, in bed, the tremor was unmistakable.

Around midnight I woke up. Unable to sleep, I turned on the bed-side radio and listened to a few minutes of a talk show about politics. Bored with the subject, I hunted around the dial until I happened upon the BBC World Broadcast. At half-past twelve, the news announcer reported an earthquake off the coast of Japan. "On Friday afternoon, 6.9 on the Richter scale."

I will concede that to construe a connection between a faint tremor in my legs and a quake off the shore of Japan suggests serious lunacy. All the same, I recorded the details in my diary and went back to sleep.

Years later, in 1989, while transcribing these notes in London, I came upon this incident in my diary, which I had forgotten. Curious as to the distance and time zones between Tokyo and Los Angeles, I rang the Information Bureau of the *London Daily Telegraph*. "Japan," they informed me, "is 16 hours ahead of Los Angeles, and the distance is roughly 5,450 miles."

I hadn't recorded the time of the tremor, but I normally ate around seven, which would be roughly noon in Japan on the following day. The quake, which occurred on Friday afternoon, was reported at 5:30 p.m. their time. If it took place within the preceding hour—say, from 4:00 to 5:00 p.m., this would have placed my symptom—if that is what it was—a few hours before.

This was the last such anomaly to occur during my four-week stay in Los Angeles. That these synchronicities happened only when I was on the Mexican-California littoral proved their origin was purely telluric. There was nothing remotely psychic about these sensations. My freakish body had simply reacted to a subtle disturbance in the earth—the way a dowser's rod reacts to an underground stream, pure or polluted, that flows beneath his feet.

I am persuaded that far more people than are aware of it experience some sort of physical change, however slight, minutes, or hours, before an earthquake, if they are within its radius—and even if they are not. If they fail to make the connection, it is simply because they lack the necessary knowledge.

The awareness is all.

On my last day at HealthMed, I saw the doctor for a checkup and review of my tests. They showed a marked reduction in the level of chemicals still in my system.

"The real test, though," I told Michael, as we said goodbye, "will be if I can reach Heathrow without having a headache on the plane."

And indeed, the flight home was headache-free, though whether because of the saunas or a stronger immune system, I cannot say. Both, I believe, contributed to this happy liberation. I do feel that saunas could be a worthy adjunct to the Gerson Therapy in treating the growing problem of environmental illness, although I would discourage anyone with a severely damaged immune system from choosing saunas as a first resort. Had I done so, I might have ended up the way Lynn did—the way Doris did too, as she told me in a letter I received two weeks after my return to London.

"I've been going downhill ever since I returned home," she wrote. "Maybe I should have stayed there longer, the way that LSD user was forced to stay in the sauna until he was clear. I don't know what I'll do now.

"By the way," she added, "I understand that shortly after you left, Mitzi dropped out of the program and returned home in high dudgeon. Some altercation with Faxon, I believe."

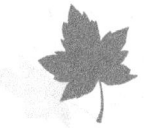

CHAPTER THIRTY-TWO

My first act on reaching home was to read *When the Snakes Awake* again in the hope of finding an explanation for the seismic synchronicities that occurred in Beverly Hills. This time, the dedication caught my eye:

> To the observers of nature without name, title or career
> for their contributions to the progress of Science.

A possible clue appeared in his chapter on the piezoelectric effect:

> If electrostatic charges do move from the ground into
> the atmosphere, and if their liberation and neutralization
> produces long electromagnetic waves and changes in the
> electric field, then sensitive people must feel the approach of
> an earthquake.

Consulting my copy of Lyall Watson's *Neophilia*, I found this passage:

> We know now that earthquakes make our whole planet ring
> like a gong, setting up long wave, low-frequency oscillations
> that go on for an hour or more and can be measured
> anywhere on earth. These vibrations occur at frequencies
> from seven to fourteen cycles per second, and the fascinating
> thing about them is that they not only accompany, but also
> precede the actual occurrence of a quake.

And in Watson's *Supernature,* referring to these low-frequency vibrations, he adds:

> These start minutes before the first obvious shocks of the quake itself and provide an early-warning system to which many species seem to respond.
>
> ... Some people, particularly women and children, are also sensitive to these frequencies. The fact that the frequencies coincide with those that make people disturbed and ill would account for the wild, unreasoning fear that goes with an earthquake.

"Wild, unreasoning fear" was precisely what I felt that last night at the clinic—yet I did not experience any premonitory fear in Los Angeles. Was it because the quakes were weaker, or because after fifteen months on the therapy I was no longer as sensitive as before?

Flare-ups now were fewer, and milder when they came, but I still had toxins to shed, so I decided to add a weekly sauna to my regime in London. Accordingly, I joined a nearby health club, but found I could not use the equipment because of the disinfectant in the gym, and I couldn't swim in the pool because of the chlorine. In the sauna, my nose recoiled from the scented lotions the women used, so I resigned from the club the same day that I joined.

Eventually, I found a less salubrious establishment where, if I arrived when it opened in the morning, I had the sauna to myself. By June, I was having two saunas a week, with detox symptoms similar to, though weaker than, those at HealthMed.

Bronya, meanwhile, having enjoyed a month's vacation in my absence, was as disputatious as ever. Resigned though I was to her labyrinthine work methods, her need to score points was beginning to get up my nose.

In February, I remarked that I was only a month away from achieving the therapy's eighteen-month milestone for cancer patients.

"Isn't it ironic, Bronya," I mused, "that having grown up in a home where meat was the focus of every meal, my health is being restored by a vegan regime that's the very opposite of my childhood diet?"

"How do you know it's not the placebo effect?" she challenged. "Maybe the therapy only works because you want it to."

"If that were so," I replied, "why didn't the other therapies I tried work as well? God knows, I wanted them to."

"But it's all in your *mind,* I tell you," she cried, with an intensity that took me off guard. "The therapy only works because you *believe* that it will!"

Too weary to wonder how a simple statement of fact had become a psychological issue, I asked her why, in that case, I had chosen the hardest therapy of all to believe in? She gave me one of her pitying little smiles, which I knew meant, "Don't blind me with logic; I've won the debate and the subject is closed."

My patience with this sort of thing had been growing thin, and in April it finally cracked. Bronya was dispatched, taking with her the day of her departure so many plastic bags filled with heaven knew what, they filled half the backseat of the cab that took her away.

Clive, in town for a meeting of the Dowsing Society on the twenty-third, arrived early to show me his latest discovery before we left for the hall. Although I was still addicted to his experiments, I was now more an observer than participant. And now that I no longer needed his help (or no longer believed that I did), our relationship was more relaxed—even playful at times.

We had already discussed the earthquake incidents in L.A., but I couldn't resist testing him again.

"Then you're quite sure, Clive, the synchronicities weren't just coincidence?"

"Oh, there's no doubt in my mind you were picking up the vibrations," he said. Few things took Clive by surprise or struck him as beyond the realm of possibility.

"Even the quakes off Alaska and Japan?"

"Of course. Given your sensitivity, I suspect you're tuned in to some sort of earthquake frequency. You're like a spider on a web, aren't you? The smallest tug at the farthest extremity of the web can still be sensed by the spider."

Not the happiest simile for an arachnophobe, but I knew what he meant. Our dowsing adventures had proven again and again the irrelevance of distance and the interconnectedness of all things. I would miss those experiments—especially the failures—for, paradoxically, it was often the failures that proved the reality of those forces that fill what we so mistakenly think of as empty space.

Bronya's successor was a forty-three-year-old American hippie, "Devla," who said she was familiar with the Norwalk juicing machine, since she had worked for a year making juices at a holistic retreat. When she added that she, too, was a vegetarian, I engaged her on the spot; at least we would be as one on the subject of nutrition.

It soon became clear, however, that what Devla *hoped* she would be doing was holding someone's hand and being "spiritual." Preparing a meal, picking up food that fell on the floor—even making the juices —was not really her thing. As slow as Bronya, and arguably more disorganized, each time she ran the juicing machine she referred to a piece of paper on which she had written the instructions.

After four difficult months, I had to tell Devla that, sadly, it was not going to work. She took it in good part, the way she seemed to take all life's vicissitudes—a quality I greatly admire and would have cherished, had it been accompanied by a modicum of efficiency.

The night before she left, Devla poked her head around the door and said, ever so winsomely, "Before I go, I just wanted you to know that my special gift is to comfort and heal. I thought I would leave that with you."

"Thank you, Devla," I said, "I appreciate your sharing that with me."

What I wanted to say was, "Your special gift may be dancing with moonbeams, but my special need is for someone to chop wood and carry water."

By August I had progressed to the modified regime with fewer juices, so I no longer needed a live-in helper. Instead, I engaged a series of foreign students who were in London to improve their English and who came for a few hours each weekday to make two juices and prepare a meal.

First came Heiki—half German, half-Spanish, and my favorite. Then came Anna—Italian, fair-haired, and studious, who helped me refresh my fading fluency in her language. Last came the Portuguese Fatima—dark, diligent, and prim. All three were such a pleasure to have around, that when the time came for each to go home, I genuinely regretted her departure. But they had better things to do with their young lives than grind vegetables for a dotty ex-pat American.

In October, I experienced a final bout of discouragement—with life, with my writing, and with the therapy, now that I was doing most of the work myself. It was hard not to feel that Someone Up There didn't want the book on adoption to be finished.

On the twenty-seventh, I moaned to my diary:

> I have never felt so discouraged. Like poor old Sisyphus I plod on year after year, setback after setback, without ever reaching my goal.
> Montaigne said he suffered from "the disease of writing books and being ashamed of them when they are finished." But his were finished. I just have the disease.

By December the picture had changed. My brain no longer felt as though it was stuffed with wool, and I was even able to undo some of the constipated prose that lay so distressingly on every page.

I also had more energy—so much, in fact, that on the fifth, I donned a track suit and jogged up the Fulham Road to the new Conran store— marveling (on the slower walk back) at how far I had run. I now realized that my problem with geopathic stress had not been caused, after all, by the fractured energy lines, real though they were, but rather by my collapsed immune system, which could have protected me from their influence.

That evening, I watched a TV show called *The Sixth Sense,* about the ability of animals to sense things of which humans are unaware.

"Scorpions in particular," said the narrator, referring to the arachnid kind, "are sensitive to air currents and are endowed with almost mystical powers that foretell earthquakes and volcanic eruptions."

Tributsch notes in his book that "Fish and aquatic animals seem to suffer more intensely from the consequences of earthquakes than do land animals."

Perhaps then, I reflected, I really was that "queer fish" Clive had so often accused me of being—not always in jest.

Five days before Christmas, I flew again, headache-free, to Los Angeles, to stay with my favorite cousin, Arlene, and her husband, Larry. I had stayed in their guest room before, enduring its perfumed scents as the price I had to pay for the fun of Arlene's company. The scents were still there, but this time I was able to tolerate them—if only just.

Temptation, however, lurked in every corner of Arlene's kitchen: In the candy-filled dish on the counter, the cartons of ice cream in the freezer, and almost everything I saw in her well-stocked refrigerator. My cousin's diet was similar to the one I was raised on: meat, fish, vegetables, lots of carbohydrates, extra salt, butter, and rich desserts. Apart from the meat, I ate everything on offer, telling myself that I had been abstinent for so long I deserved a proper binge.

Larry, a doctor, was addicted to Diet Pepsi and spooned lecithin granules onto his cereal each morning. When he died of Alzheimer's in his seventies, I wondered if the aspartame in the colas might have contributed to the disease.

On the afternoon of January 2, I felt fatigued and went to bed early that evening. Shortly after midnight, I woke with a parched throat and the familiar tingling in my feet. Since my fingers, too, were throbbing and had turned bright red, I attributed these symptoms to my many dietary infractions.

The next morning, while rummaging in the kitchen for something I could eat, I turned on the radio. I was sectioning a grapefruit when the news came on:

> There has been a small earthquake six miles southeast of Pasadena, 3.2 on the Richter scale.

At dinner that evening, my feet began to quiver under the table. Towards midnight I woke with another mild headache and that tiny motor starting up in the sole of each foot. The next day there was an aftershock of the Pasadena quake in Orange County.

These were the last such disturbances that occurred during my visit home. They were also the last of my "premonitory" symptoms.

In 1990, after twenty happy years in England, I returned to California to be near my daughters and settled in Santa Barbara, because I didn't want to live in Beverly Hills again. When the Northridge earthquake struck in January 1994—at 6.7 the worst quake in the Los Angeles basin since 1971—the only physical anomaly I thought worth recording the day before was a vague feeling of illness.

With this proof that I was no longer that spider on a web, "trembling at the slightest tug from the farthest extremity," I realized that at long last my immune system had been restored.

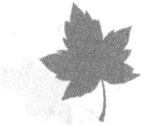

CHAPTER THIRTY-THREE

M y return to California after thirty-two years abroad was only partially successful. Had it not been for the sea, the Santa Barbara Writers' Conference each year, and work on my book, I would have missed my life in London even more than I did.

In 1996 a friend invited me to visit her in North Carolina. The only thing I knew about the state was that it was the home of the Rhine Research Center, where J.B. Rhine pioneered the science of parapsychology at Duke University in the 1930s. I had learned about the Rhine when I was trying to get rid of the poltergeist in our flat. I never imagined I would live in the south one day, but when I saw the glorious foliage—the dogwoods and crape myrtles—coupled with the dual proximity of mountains and beaches, the cleanliness of the state and the friendliness of the people—not to mention the presence of the Rhine, it had a kind of just-rightness to it, and I felt it was where I belonged.

In 1999, I needed another operation on my toes; they hadn't healed properly because of my earlier refusal of the pins. Now, however, fifteen years had passed and I was no longer as sensitive to "inert" matter as before.

My new foot surgeon could not have been more congenial or less like his odious predecessor in London. Sandy-haired and smiling, Dr. Hauser examined my feet and explained that in order to correct the problem, he would need to put a pin in each toe. I told him about my previous experience and expressed my concern.

Instead of the dismissive response I expected, he handed me a leaflet saying, "This will explain some of the postoperative reactions you might have." On opening it, the first words I saw were, "You may have an allergic reaction to the steel pins or the nylon sutures."

Well, well, I thought, podiatry has come a long way since 1985—at least on this side of the pond. Delighted to have found a doctor who was not only sympathetic, but informed, I decided this time to risk the pins. I was still apprehensive about the postoperative pain, however, the memory of that night in the hospital having been etched into my cortex.

The morning of the operation, I declined the nurse's offer of a pre-op Valium "to calm your nerves," since I had no nerves that needed to be calmed. When I came to in the recovery room she asked, "Would you like something to drink? A Coke? Ginger Ale? Water? Or something to eat? Graham crackers? Saltines?" I accepted the water, having prepared oatmeal and fruit for when I returned home.

To my surprise, I needed only one painkiller that day, and now that my toes were pinned I had no need of a cast, only a funny-looking shoe and the help of a walker for the first few days. Indeed, the whole experience would have been problem-free, had it not been for my own stupidity. Dr. Hauser had instructed me to stay in bed with an ice pack on my raised foot. However, the day after the surgery, I had been up with the walker for much of the time due to an unusual number of visitors.

First came the gardener, who needed to know where to plant the cherry tree. Next came the heating engineer to fix a problem with the thermostat. Then a member of my writing group came to collect my critique of her story for the meeting that night, which I could not attend. Last came a "friend" who wanted to go over some documents that were to be placed in my safe deposit box at the bank. This could have waited for weeks, but, as I realized only later, her sense of urgency was because one of the documents was my will and she was a beneficiary. Instead of staying in bed as I should have done, I sat with her on the sofa while we went through the papers together. It did strike me as odd that she scarcely noticed my condition—but then her concerns lay elsewhere.

When Dr. Hauser rang that evening to see how I was doing, I had to admit that I'd been on my feet a bit that day.

"You mean you haven't been staying in bed with your foot raised?"

"No," I confessed, "and my toes are bleeding quite a lot, but I suppose that's normal."

"No, it is not," he said, sharply. "That will increase the swelling. You should have stayed in bed with an ice pack on your toes."

I felt suitably chastened. As a result of this infraction my toes bled profusely, their healing was delayed—and the "friend" is no longer in my life.

On the twenty-seventh I saw Dr. Hauser to have my blood-soaked dressing changed.

"Due to the excessive bleeding," he said, "I'm going to have to put you on antibiotics for ten days to prevent infection."

"Oh, no!" I cried. "Not *more* antibiotics—just when I've spent two years getting rid of the old ones!"

On the sixth of October Dr. Hauser removed the stitches from my toes—so gently that I scarcely felt a thing.

"You seem to be tolerating the pins quite well," he observed.

The difference between this experience and the one in London was so marked that if I hadn't been for fear of alarming him, I would have leapt off the table and given Dr. Hauser a hug.

By the twelfth, however, I began to feel a familiar pressure building up in my toes. Suspecting the pins, I realized that although I had managed to tolerate them for four weeks, I couldn't have done so indefinitely.

"I can see you're reacting to the pins," said Dr. Hauser, when we met two days later, "because there's a bit more swelling here than there should be."

Within moments of his removing the pins—a distinctly painful procedure this time—the relief was palpable. By the time I was heading home, my toes felt as though they had just bathed in a cool, soothing stream.

The discovery that my body could still not accept a foreign substance for any length of time suggested to me that once an immune system has been compromised, the need for caution remains. Whether our bodies were meant to cope with an ever more toxic environment I will leave for future generations to decide.

While discussing this vestigial sensitivity with Dr. Hauser during a follow-up visit, he told me about another patient on whose foot he had operated.

"When her leg began to swell inside the cast—I think it was two months after the operation—I decided to remove the screw. Even before it was completely out, she said, 'Oh, that feels so much better!' And another patient reacted to the soluble sutures, which kept rising to the surface of her skin. I would cut off the bit that stuck out, only to have the rest of the suture slowly emerge and need to be cut off as well."

Shades of that rhinoplasty patient again.

"So you see," he added, with an engaging grin, "you're not the only patient whose body has tried to reject a foreign object."

Oh, if only someone had told me that years ago, I thought, what pain I could have been spared!

Three weeks later, while examining my foot at my final checkup, Dr. Hauser was surprised to find he had overlooked a suture in one toe.

Had he not told me it was there, I would never have known.

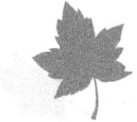

CHAPTER THIRTY-FOUR

Max Gerson's achievement was not that he found a cure for cancer in the 1930s, but that he developed a nutritional therapy that restores the body's immune system, enabling it to correct whatever is out of balance, be it cancer, lupus, or a migraine headache.[3]

When Hippocrates wrote, "Let food be your medicine, let your medicine be your food," he did not mean the processed, denatured, tarted-up artifact that we call "food" today. Overfed and undernourished, we have surrendered our well-being to the food industry whose lure of "convenience food" means whatever is most convenient (and profitable) for them, not what is healthiest for us. It is not convenient to have cancer. It is not convenient to have a bulimic child. It is not convenient to waste money on pills and potions in an attempt to replace the natural, life-giving nutrients we have destroyed through synthetic preparation.

Our palates have become so jaded that unless we eat organically, we no longer know what real food tastes like. Meanwhile, our fast foods are taking us ever more swiftly toward an earlier grave. As Michael Pollan observes in his book *In Defense of Food,* "What people *don't* eat may matter as much as what they do."

We are told that fractional amounts of chemicals in our food do not cause us harm. Yet fractions accumulate, interacting with all the other toxins we are exposed to, and with consequences that no one can foresee. Add to these all the pharmaceutical and recreational drugs we consume, it is no wonder that some of us are turning into toxic time bombs.

3 See the complete list of contraindications and cautions for the Gerson Therapy online at gerson.org.

The function of food is not to titillate our taste buds or bloat our bellies, but to nourish each cell of the complex structure that serves as our only vehicle in this lifetime. That function is now endangered by genetically modified (GMO) food, the long-term safety of which has not been proved. Those who wish to avoid GMO food cannot do so unless it is labeled as such. By refusing to label, the Food and Drug Administration is protecting Monsanto, not the consumer.

In 2009, President Obama appointed Michael R. Taylor, a former lobbyist for Monsanto, as a senior adviser to the FDA Commissioner on Food Safety. As a high-ranking official at the FDA in the '90s, Taylor had promoted the introduction of genetically modified organisms into the US food supply without the requirement of a single safety test. He also allowed the agency to ignore evidence that GM foods, including soy, were very different from natural foods and posed specific health risks.

In 1997, the FDA changed its rules to allow widespread advertising of prescription drugs directly to consumers. In 2004, the pharmaceutical industry spent over four hundred million dollars on TV and radio commercials, print ads, and Web-based promotions. Today, it is more like *eight* hundred million dollars. Five hundred million dollars was spent on Vioxx® alone before a study confirmed that the arthritis drug raised the risk of heart attacks and stroke and it was finally pulled from the market. The public, of course, pays for these ad campaigns through the grossly inflated prices of prescription drugs.

Commercials are about making money, not about curing disease, and all such advertising should be banned. A pill that relieves your headache may be concealing the cause, which could be a food allergy, a swollen blood vessel, or a brain tumor. Acid indigestion and heartburn are not telling you to take an antacid, they are warning you to change your diet.

Spoiled by surfeit and strangers to self-denial, we've become addicted to the quick fix: Got a headache, backache, constipation, indigestion, spotty skin, sexual hang-up, smokers' cough, bad breath? Take this pill for instant, soothing relief: the American Way of Health. But is health the result? No matter, it beats dealing with the cause, which could mean having to give up something, such as the sugar-laden goodies the next commercial will be urging us to buy.

One radio ad boasted of the drugs a pharmaceutical company had developed for children with so-called ailments such as hyperactivity. "It's the benefits of pharmaceutical research that sustain the hope of Americans for the best in health care," said the spokesman. No mention of the side effects of Ritalin®, Paxil®, Prozac®, and other psychotropic drugs.

Psychiatrist Peter Breggin points out that Eric Harris, one of the Columbine killers, had been seeing a psychiatrist and was on the antidepressant Luvox® at the time of the shooting. And Andreas Lubitz, the copilot who deliberately flew a Germanwings plane into the French Alps, killing 150 people, was afterwards found to have been taking antidepressants for a condition he kept secret.

Why does the FDA approve drugs with such dangerous side effects while labeling as "controversial" those methods that are safe and successful?

Drug companies pay doctors millions of dollars to promote their drugs at conferences. A preponderance of these doctors are psychiatrists, who can earn as much as $500,000 or more for their endorsement. How objective can a doctor be when selecting your treatment, if he is receiving thousands of dollars from a drug maker?

A recent cartoon showed two doctors strolling down a hospital corridor, one saying to the other:

"I have no objection to alternative medicine so long as traditional medical fees are scrupulously maintained."

A drug can be on the market for years before its dangers are confirmed, by which time thousands of people will have been injured or died. Vioxx® and Zyprexa® were not withdrawn until years after they had been in widespread use, and Zoloft®, Paxil®, and Prozac® had been out for more than a decade before black-box warnings of "suicidal behavior" were finally added. It took the FDA 35 years to warn that acetaminophen can damage the liver, and the sweetener aspartame has been on the market since 1996.

All drugs should be judged guilty until proven innocent!

In 2011, the Archives of Internal Medicine published a scathing re-assessment of a flawed twelve-year-old research study of Neurontin®, an anti-seizure drug, made by Pfizer. Eleven patients in the study died and 73 experienced "serious adverse events." Had *one* patient died as a result of alternative treatment, the media and the medical boards would have been braying for the therapist's head.

Medical pioneers like Gerson face the same persecution today that every visionary has faced who dared to defy entrenched opinion. The forces that oppose them are also the same. They are massive, powerful, and rich—like the $235 million Cancer Center Duke University opened in Durham, North Carolina, in 2012.

"Covering 267,000 square feet," reads the dedication announcement, the Center "has radiology services, radiation oncology, a mammography suite, and three new linear accelerators. It also has 73 infusion stations where 120 patients can receive chemotherapy each day, not to mention a specialty pharmacy so that patients can fill their prescriptions on site."

As Deepak Chopra observed, "More people *live* off cancer than die of it."

"More than 600 cancer patients are currently seen daily in Duke clinics," continues the announcement. *"New cancer cases in North Carolina are projected to grow by 16.5 percent in five years."*

Really? What, then, became of all those promising breakthroughs we've been reading about for years that were going to reduce the incidence of cancer? When the next breakthrough is announced, I suggest we ask the following questions:

- Who paid for the research?

- What aspect of the study is being withheld?

- What further research needs to be done?

- What proof of its efficacy do you have *now*—not in animal studies, but in human beings?

Meanwhile, in 2013, when the country was facing a deficit of more than \$1.2 trillion and automatic spending cuts were being widely imposed, Duke University School of Medicine—one of the richest institutions in America—was receiving \$417 million in taxpayers' money from the National Institutes of Health to keep researchers searching for a cure for cancer.

In the words of Krishnamurti:

> *It is no measure of health to be well-adjusted to a profoundly sick society.*

CHAPTER THIRTY-FIVE

When I began this account of my search for health some years ago, the journey was still in progress and its conclusion was far from certain. Although I now have a restored immune system, and geopathic stress is a distant nightmare, I still wished there could be an easier method than Gerson's for those who find his regime too difficult to follow. After all, no one approach works for everyone, and in some cases genetic predisposition limits the curative options.

In January 2010, the chance came to test a simpler method when a small lump in my breast was diagnosed as non-Hodgkin's lymphoma. My nice GP, who indulges my eccentricities, told me not to worry—he would start me immediately on chemotherapy. I thanked him, but said I would go instead to Houston to see Dr. Burzynski. If my GP thought I was mad, he was much too polite to say so.

Dr. Stanislaw Burzynski is a Polish-born doctor who has over forty years' experience in treating cancer. He earned both his medical degree and a Ph.D. in biochemistry before he was 24—a rare achievement—and graduated "with distinction" at the top of his science class in Poland.

While doing research at Baylor College of Medicine in Houston, Texas, Burzynski discovered "antineoplastons." These are components of the body's biochemical defense against cancer that act as "molecular switches," turning on tumor suppressor genes and turning off oncogenes. In 1977, he resigned from the college and established Burzynski Research Laboratories in order to manufacture his patented discovery.

In addition to his treatment for cancer, Burzynski has discovered new treatments for autoimmune diseases, viral infections, Parkinson's disease, neurofibromatosis, restenosis, and AIDS. He has over 242 patents from 42 countries and has contributed to over 300 scientific publications.

His path in this country, however, has been far from smooth. Although initially his research was sponsored by the National Cancer Institute, he has since incurred the wrath of the entire cancer establishment. Why? Because he proved his antineoplastons (ANPs) cured cancers that his colleagues had said were incurable—and did so without the harmful side effects of their drugs.

In FDA-permitted Phase II trials for inoperable brain tumors, Burzynski's ANPs achieved more than five years' survival in 122 cases—all of whom had failed standard treatments. Notwithstanding his proven success, he was still required to go through a Phase III trial to obtain FDA approval. However, since he received no grants, he lacked the forty million dollars needed to fund the trial and without FDA approval, his treatment could not be covered by insurance. The patients, moreover, would be first required to go through the standard of care treatment, which means they would need to fail both chemo and radiation before being allowed to have antineoplastons. In other words, their immune systems would have to be destroyed *before* Burzynski could try to cure them.

In the 1980s and '90s, the FDA launched—and lost—three litigations against Dr. Burzynski. At each of these trials, a significant number of his cured cancer patients traveled to Washington to testify on his behalf. (See the documentary *Burzynski, Cancer Is a Serious Business*.)

Thus, a government agency spent sixty million dollars of taxpayers' money trying to put a cancer-curing doctor out of business. At the same time, newspaper headlines were warning that contaminated fish were being sold in grocery stores and restaurants, which the FDA claimed it lacked the resources to inspect.

In February 2012, when the country was experiencing a shortage of cancer drugs, the FDA announced that it would allow the import of generic drugs made in India. The quality of drugs from India is notoriously unreliable, there being no systematic oversight in that country. At the same time the FDA refused to let Dr. Burzynski provide his antineoplastons, large amounts of which he could have manufactured in his own laboratory, which is regularly inspected by the FDA and kept to the highest standards.

Why are drugs hailed as merely hopeful given prime-time publicity by the mainstream media, while Burzynski's proven success is repeatedly ignored? The answer is simple: because the media's revenue depends largely on its pharmaceutical advertising.

The persecution of Dr. Burzynski began in 1983, when the FDA filed a lawsuit against him in the federal courts in Houston. The Texas Medical Board began its action in 1984. It asked Burzynski to present 20 cases of cancer patients who were treated with his antineoplastons; if it found the patients had received any benefit, the Board would leave him alone. Burzynski presented not 20 but 40 cases, each one showing remarkable improvement. The Board then went back on its agreement and has been harassing him ever since. For 30 years the TMB has known that antineoplastons can cure terminal cancers, yet it is still trying to put Burzynski out of business. As a result of its efforts, untold cancer victims whose lives could have been saved have died.

The facts, briefly, are these:

- In the 1980s, Burzynski successfully completed the first investigative new trial of antineoplastons for inoperable brain tumors. Only patients deemed incurable after standard treatments had failed were allowed to participate in the trial. The National Cancer Institute (NCI) reviewed seven of the brain tumor cases and decided to fund Phase II trials.

- These trials—for anaplastic astrocytomas—were held between March 1988 and December 1989. At the same time, an agreement was signed between Dr. Burzynski and Elan Pharmaceuticals, according to which Elan would organize and fund clinical trials that would lead to FDA approval of antineoplastons.

- Four patients in this trial obtained complete remission; two patients had more than 50% decrease of the tumor size, and ten patients obtained stabilization of the disease. Seven patients had a marked decrease of the tumor size, and four patients developed progressive disease. Two of the patients, alive at this writing, have been tumor-free for over 20 years.

- When Elan learned the details of the Phase II trial, it reneged on its agreement with Burzynski, intending to reproduce his results on its own by using one of the ingredients in antineoplastons, sodium phenylacetate (PN). Elan then obtained the cooperation of Dr. Dvorit Samid, who worked for Burzynski, and who then agreed to be employed by the National Cancer Institute.

- To fund its own clinical trial with phenylacetate, Elan donated $15 million to NCI. However, antineoplastons contain two additional ingredients that are more important than PN. The clinical trials NCI had promised Burzynski were postponed for four years in order to let Elan complete its own trial. When the trial failed, as was expected, Elan, NCI, and Dr. Samid decided to separate antineoplaston therapy from its creator—the word "separate" being their euphemism for "steal."

- In 1994, NCI finally started a single trial with ANPs, but to ensure the trial would fail, they used a dose 50 times smaller than the one required. In 1995, Burzynski's attorney had to force NCI to stop the "low-dose" trial, in order to save the patients' lives.

- A friend of Elan, Michael A. Friedman, who was in charge of the NCI project, then moved to the FDA to become the Deputy Commissioner. Shortly thereafter, a grand jury indicted Dr. Burzynski. Dr. Friedman was aware of the TMB's parallel action because Burzynski had told him about it and asked for his help, which Friedman refused.

- The FDA and NCI knew that Burzynski received no grants and that his main income came from his private practice. Thus, if the TMB could place a restriction on his practice, Burzynski would be deprived of financial resources and therefore have no means of defending himself.

- Elan, the NCI, and Dr. Samid then "appropriated" Dr. Burzynski's patent. The only way they could use it, however, was if Burzynski could be put in prison. The cooperation of the Texas Medical Board, therefore, was essential.

Ironically, had Burzynski remained in Poland, he would have had more freedom to practice medicine than he has found here in America, our "Land of the Free".

For those of us who owe our lives to alternative therapies, mistrust of the FDA began in July 1985, when its agents entered the clinics of a number of alternative practitioners and proceeded to search them, even though Amendment IV of the Constitution states: "The right of the people to be secure in their persons, houses, papers, and effects, against unreasonable searches and seizures, shall not be violated...."

The agents seized eleven of Dr. Burzynski's filing cabinets, which contained his patients' private medical records and all his billing and insurance files. Some of the supplement manufacturers who were also raided could not afford the cost of defending themselves and were put out of business—which, of course, was the intent.

That the motive behind these raids was not to protect the public, but to protect the pharmaceutical companies is borne out by one of the stated goals of the "Dietary Supplements Task Force Final Report" of May 1992:

TO ENSURE THAT THE EXISTENCE OF DIETARY SUPPLEMENTS ON THE MARKET DOES NOT ACT AS A DISINCENTIVE FOR DRUG DEVELOPMENT.

Such raids increased in the 1990s when David Kessler became commissioner of the agency. Doctors' offices were invaded by Special Weapons and Tactics (SWAT) teams with drawn guns, who confiscated medical equipment and patients' confidential files on the pretext that methods were being used which the FDA had not approved.[4]

And why had approval been withheld? Not because a single patient had died or been injured, as have thousands on FDA-approved Vioxx®, Paxil®, Avastin®, and other such drugs, but because the legitimate practice of safe, alternative therapies poses an economic threat to the obscene profits of the pharmaceutical companies.

In his book *The Rise of Tyranny*, Jonathan Emord records how, in the '90s, Kessler refused to allow a *proven* claim associating folic acid with a reduction in the risk of neural tube defect births to appear on dietary supplements containing the product. By disallowing that claim, Emord writes, Kessler contributed to an estimated 2,500 children a year being born with spina bifida or anencephaly, all of which could have been prevented.

Note: In February 2015, Kessler was a guest on an NPR program about vitamins and supplements. Asked whether he thought they should be regulated, he said:

> "There is so much we don't know about them. We know they work in certain circumstances. I worked hard to fortify the food supply with folic acid so that pregnant women could

4 Dr. Jonathan Wright. *FDA vs. The People of the United States: Five years of assault on "self care."* 1995.

avoid giving birth to children with neural tube defects. We have reduced the incidence of this defect. It's one of the things I'm proudest of."

In a speech Kessler gave to a small group of journalists in March 1996, he announced a fast track for approving cancer drugs that were "promising in Europe. The FDA will approve them now," he said, "and test them later." Most of these were "me, too" drugs—no better, and often worse than those already on the market, whose relative safety, at least, had been tested over time.

"We want to provide accelerated access to drugs that *work!*" he said.

"What about antineoplastons?" asked one of the journalists.

"I'm talking about science," said Kessler without missing a beat, as though Burzynski was not a scientist. "Politics plays no part in this decision," he added—a curious disclaimer from one who has worked for much of his life as an administrative bureaucrat.

Another nonpracticing doctor who joined the attacks on Burzynski in the 1990s used his radio program to spread the FDA's discredited charges against him. This former ophthalmologist—who admitted he quit medicine because it bored him—also claimed that successful alternative cures were due to "the placebo effect," even though babies and animals, who are immune to autosuggestion, respond to homeopathic treatment.

Sifting through medical journals in the comfort of his office or his home, this former eye doctor became far wealthier by denigrating the achievements of others than he could have become by trying to cure cancer himself. Of course, by attacking Burzynski, he kept his sponsors happy, his listeners in ignorance, and his multimillion-dollar lifestyle assured.

"Great spirits have always encountered violent opposition from mediocre minds," observed Einstein.

One brave doctor who fought the establishment's attempts to discredit him was the late Dr. Nicholas J. Gonzalez of New York City, who died suddenly in July 2015 at the age of 67. His protocol was similar to Gerson's in that it, too, stressed organic nutrition, enzymes, coffee enemas, and other means of detoxification.

In 2005, Dr. Gonzalez learned that the American Cancer Society had just printed six million pamphlets attacking Burzynski, Gerson, and himself. A man of strong character, he threatened to sue the ACS if it dared to distribute its scurrilous propaganda. Knowing that its lies could not have stood up in a court of law, the ACS had to trash every one of the six million pamphlets.

And this, donors, is how the American Cancer Society spends your money.

Pioneering doctors like Gerson, Burzynski, and others before them, have risked losing their licenses and their livelihoods for being in advance of their times.

"In science," wrote Sir William Osler, "the credit goes to the man who convinces the world, not to the man to whom the idea first occurs."

As for the small tumor found in my breast in 2010, an MRI in 2013 revealed that it had shrunk to a 0.6 cm mass after Burzynski's treatment. A year later, my final MRI showed the mass to be stable, with no lymph node involvement.

Had I been able to have antineoplastons, I'm sure the tumor could have been gone within a year.

CHAPTER THIRTY-SIX

Tori Moreno was born in 1998 with a tumor occupying her entire brainstem. Diffuse intrinsic pontine (brainstem) gliomas (DIPG) are inoperable and carry the worst prognosis in the oncology field. Told by their oncologist the tumor was inoperable and the child would not see her first birthday, the distraught parents asked if he knew of any other option they could try. He said he did not.

Turning to the Internet, they discovered Dr. Burzynski and appealed to him as a last resort. When she was brought to the clinic, Tori had been given only one month to live. Dr. Burzynski told the parents he had never treated a child that young so he could make no promises, but the baby was given his antineoplastons and her tumor began to shrink.

The parents' medical insurance, however, did not cover unorthodox treatments. When their funds ran low, they begged the insurance company to help with the payments, which it would have done for surgery, chemo, or a bone marrow transplant—all three riskier, more costly, and more painful procedures.

Because of Tori's improvement, their provider agreed—on condition that the parents accept a gag order. They were not to disclose the insurance company's involvement, nor could they speak publicly of the therapy that was saving their baby's life. The company would not even deal directly with Burzynski, but arranged for payment to be made through the parents.

At the end of eight months Tori was in remission. Today she is a healthy young girl of seventeen, one of the many children with terminal cancers whose lives "Dr. B." has saved. (Some time after her treatment, her parents learned that their oncologist had known about Burzynski when he said there were no other options.)

David Emerson was 34 when he was diagnosed with multiple myeloma in February 1994. He underwent induction therapy of 5 rounds of VAD (vincristine, Adriamycin®, dexamethasone), 2 rounds of Cytoxan®, and an autologous bone marrow transplant, all in 1995. In October '96 he relapsed, underwent local palliative radiation to reduce the pain in his bones, relapsed again in September '97, and was told "nothing more can be done for you."

On learning that the Burzynski clinic was holding clinical trials, he went to Houston. The trials were for inoperable brain tumors, but because David had an atypical form of multiple myeloma, the FDA made an exception for him on the grounds of "compassionate use."

David began intravenous antineoplaston therapy in November '97. Radiological evaluation was required every eight weeks—either CT scan or MRI—as were monthly visits with his local doctor and periodic visits to the clinic, about every four months. By April '99 he had achieved complete remission and remains cancer-free to this day.

His only suffering has been from the long-term, late-stage side effects of his conventional cancer treatment. These conditions include chemo-induced peripheral neuropathy, radiation-induced lumbosacral plexopathy, chemo-induced heart damage resulting in chronic atrial fibrillation, irritable bladder, and "chemo-brain" (post-chemo cognitive impairment).

Thomas Navarro's story, sadly, has a different ending. At the age of four, Thomas was diagnosed with a medulloblastoma, a type of brain tumor that, if untreated, has few survivors. Treatment, however, can cause numerous side effects, including extreme mental disability. Following surgery the oncologist proposed chemotherapy with radiation to the brain. Unwilling to subject their son to the risks of further invasive treatment, the Navarros decided to look for alternative answers on the Internet. (See the documentary *Cut, Poison, and Burn,* cutpoisonburn. com/.) Finding Dr. Burzynski's name connected with successful brain tumor treatment, they took Thomas to Houston.

When they told their doctor they were seeking another opinion and would try Dr. Burzynski's treatment, the doctor, without their knowledge, notified the Child Protective Services. CPS tried to take Thomas away from the Navarros on charges of child cruelty and neglect. At the same time, they were told by the FDA that in order to see Burzynski, Thomas would first have to go through chemo and radiation, fail both, and have measurable tumors before he would be allowed to have antineoplastons. The Navarros refused to accept such a condition. Having served in the military as an Emergency Department nurse, Donna Navarro had seen firsthand the toxic consequences of chemotherapy and radiation.

For two and a half years the Navarros fought the FDA and CPS, a struggle that left them physically exhausted and financially ruined. Jim Navarro tells of meeting with a member of Congress at the time who warned him to back off, saying "Son, you can't go there. You're going to cost a lot of people a lot of money, put a lot of people out of work, and they're just not going to take kindly to that. You'll never live to see him treated. Back off."

By the time they received permission to take Thomas to Burzynski, it was too late. He had developed 50 tumors throughout his brain and spine and had been given two weeks to live. Nonetheless, Thomas began antineoplaston therapy on April 13, 2001. Although the tumors began to shrink and his life was extended for another seven months, he died on November 18 of that year. The Navarros are convinced that had Thomas been able to start the treatment before his body was poisoned by chemicals, he would be alive today.

The long struggle to save their son cost the Navarros everything they had, eventually including their marriage. When Thomas died, they were deeply in debt and had another four-year-old to care for. They were homeless, with $4 between them, and were living out of their van.

That a government agency—the so-called Child *Protective* Services— can take a child away from caring parents simply because they refuse to subject him to painful orthodox treatment should be a matter of grave concern to us all.

Our Constitution forbids any law that impinges on the rights of its citizens, yet a group of bureaucrats in Washington, beholden to the pharmaceutical industry, has assumed the power of life or death over us all. We now have a government that forbids life-saving treatment for the terminally ill who want desperately to live, while forbidding compassionate suicide for the terminally ill who want desperately to die. The law forbids cruel and inhumane punishment for the criminal, but condemns the innocent victim with a terminal disease to years of unspeakable agony.

To tell a person with motor neuron disease that they must endure the gradual shutdown of every bodily function until they are slowly choking to death is moral sadism. Physician-assisted suicide is not a cry for help; it is a cry for release when all hope of help is gone.

The British physician Lord Horder, referring to the Hippocratic Oath, said, "It is the duty of a doctor to prolong life, but it is not his duty to prolong the act of dying."

In January 2009, a group of physicians and scientists at the Food and Drug Administration wrote a letter to John D. Podesta at the Department of Health and Human Services, charging rampant corruption at the agency and pleading that it be reformed.

"There is an atmosphere at FDA in which the honest employee fears the dishonest employee, and not the other way around," they wrote. "Those committed to integrity and the FDA mission cannot act without fear of reprisal."

Citing examples of "shocking managerial corruption, wrongdoing and retaliation throughout the agency," they added, "We desperately need *honesty without fear of retaliation* for our evaluations and recommendations, as well as for accountability and transparency to become law. The long-standing FDA practice of secret meetings and secret communications between FDA managers and regulated industry must be strictly prohibited."

And nothing was done.

Among the examples of wrongdoing cited by the whistle-blowers were:

- Receiving written threats of disciplinary action if physicians and scientists failed to change their scientific opinions and recommendations to conform to those of management

- Being ordered by the director of the Office of Device Evaluation (ODE) to ignore FDA Guidance documents

- Removing Black Box warnings recommended by FDA experts

- Excluding FDA experts from participating in panel meetings because manufacturers "expressed concerns that [FDA experts] are biased"

The writers called for the removal and punishment of all managers who had participated in the well-documented corruption. For *seven* months, they stated, the commissioner and his "assistant commissioner for accountability and integrity" had conducted a sham investigation, at the end of which no one was held accountable, and no appropriate actions were taken. The same managers who had engaged in these offenses remained in place. They were even rewarded and promoted, while those who'd had the courage to speak out and had refused to comply with the wrongdoing had suffered ongoing retaliation.

The whole agency was riddled with conflicts of interest, they wrote, with many of the FDA's advisors *working as consultants for the drug companies.*

A case in point: Of the six members of the advisory committee that in 1999 recommended approving Vioxx®—the arthritis drug that was withdrawn in 2004 because it caused heart attacks—four had received waivers from the conflict-of-interest rule.

Six years after a biomedical engineer had filed a lawsuit against the FDA, a judge concluded that "the independent facts confirm the longstanding pandemic corruption that cries out for new leadership at FDA from the bottom up."

And yet, nothing was done.

In 2007, Marcia Angell, a physician and former editor-in-chief of the *New England Journal of Medicine,* wrote in an article for the *Boston Globe,* "It's time to take the Food and Drug Administration back from the drug companies."

Pointing out that in 1992 Congress passed the Prescription Drug User Fee Act, which authorizes drug companies to pay "user fees" to the FDA for each brand-name drug considered for approval, Dr. Angell observed that, "In effect, this put the FDA on the payroll of the industry it regulates. Last year, the fees came to about $300 million, which the companies recover many times over by getting their drugs to market more quickly and charging exorbitant prices.

"But while it's a small investment for the drug companies, it's a lot of money for the agency, and it has drastically changed the way it operates—creating a disproportionate emphasis on approving brand-name drugs in a hurry. Consequently, the part of the agency that reviews new drugs gets more than half its money from user fees—and it has grown rapidly, while the parts that monitor safety, ensure manufacturing standards, and check ads for accuracy have languished or even shrunk.

"The FDA now behaves as though the pharmaceutical industry is its user, not the public," she added, and concludes: "It is simply no longer possible to believe much of the clinical research that is published, or to rely on the judgment of trusted physicians or authoritative medical guidelines. I take no pleasure in this conclusion, which I reached slowly and reluctantly over my two decades as an editor of the *New England Journal of Medicine.*"

And still, nothing has changed.

Sixty years ago, the FDA was a very different agency. Its finest hour was in 1960 when Frances Kelsey, a newly appointed FDA physician, blocked approval of the drug thalidomide because it was suspected of causing phocomelia—a condition that causes babies to be born with shortened limbs, flipper-like appendages for hands or feet, or no limbs at all. A potent and inadequately tested teratogen, thalidomide was sold in the '50s and '60s chiefly to pregnant women to combat morning sickness.

Bravely resisting pressure from its German manufacturer for a swift approval of the drug, Dr. Kelsey refused, thereby sparing America the deformities with which 10,000 children in forty-six other countries were born. Most of the women who took thalidomide escaped giving birth to deformed babies, but in the game of chemical roulette, the odds against escape are often shorter.

"I cannot believe that God plays dice with the universe," said Einstein. Yet that is precisely what the FDA is doing with our health—and doing so, moreover, with a god-like arrogance.

The agency needs to be reminded that the initials FDA stand for Food and Drug Administration—not Food, Drug and *Doctor* Administration. It should be stripped of its dictatorial power and confined to the job for which it was formed: to ensure the purity of our food and the safety of our drugs.

That is all.

CHAPTER THIRTY-SEVEN

J'ACCUSE

I accuse the Food and Drug Administration of gross inhumanity and abuse of its power. I accuse the Agency of protecting Big Pharma while denying victims access to the drug-free therapies that could save their lives.

I accuse the American Medical Association of branding as "frauds" doctors whose discoveries threaten the massive profits of the pharmaceutical industry, because its ads subsidize the Journal of the AMA.

I accuse the American Cancer Society and the National Cancer Institute of defaming those doctors who cure cancer without drugs. And who sits on the Board of Directors of the ACS? Why, executives and employees of the drug industries, of course.

I accuse the Susan G. Komen Breast Cancer Foundation of hypocrisy. The cures of Gerson and Burzynski are known to them, yet the Komen Foundation gives millions of dollars to researchers each year so they can "search for a cure for breast cancer"—a *chemical* cure, that is.

I accuse the mainstream media of dereliction of duty by refusing to report the truth about successful drug-free cures. I accuse the media of dishonesty—as much for the facts it leaves out of a story as for the bias it puts in.

I accuse James Randi of using his "education foundation" not to educate, but to destroy Dr. Stanislaw Burzynski. Dr. Burzynski is a cancer-curing scientist. Randi, a former magician, is a self-promoting showman.

I accuse Randi and his "skeptics" of cyberbullying. In 2013 they attacked the Burzynski Patient Group website, flooding it with hundreds of fake emails for weeks so that genuine cancer victims seeking help and information could not get through. Not only did they disable the website, they subjected its volunteer creator—a grateful patient who was cured of stage four non-Hodgkin's lymphoma in 1993—to unremitting torment.

As an added touch, Randi's "skeptics" sent Burzynski a nasty card on his birthday.

Nice people.

Why has this doctor been singled out for such relentless attack? Has he harmed a single patient, as others have done with impunity? No. What, then, is his crime? He has dared to cure terminal cancers that his colleagues have said were incurable—and to do so, moreover, with his own patented medicine.

In announcing the creation of his "foundation" Randi wrote:

"The Foundation is generously funded by a sponsor in Washington, D.C., who wishes, at this point in time, to remain anonymous."

Might that sponsor be connected to the pharmaceutical industry by chance? And should the sponsors of tax-free foundations be allowed to conceal their affiliations? Does the IRS know that this 501(c)(3) foundation is spending millions of our dollars trying to destroy a scientist who has dedicated his life to curing cancer?

Why are such hate-filled people being supported by your tax dollars and mine, under the guise of a foundation dedicated to education?

In 2007, Randi's official salary was listed as $200,000 a year, but he receives many thousands more in "dark money" from contributors whose identities he is not required to disclose. According to page 15, line 13 of the Foundation's tax report from 2007 to 2011, its "total support" came to $5,618,789.

Not bad for a former magician. Dr. Burzynski can't afford a Phase III clinical trial.

Our country was founded on freedom, and for all its faults it has upheld that vision, even when the vision was being betrayed.

Freedom of religion is enshrined in our Constitution; blacks won their freedom from slavery in 1863; women won the right to vote in 1920 and their right to abortion in 1973. Even same-sex couples have won their right to marry, yet our right to freedom of choice in medical treatment is still being denied. Why? Because it threatens the power and profits of a multibillion-dollar medical monopoly.

The issue is not just Burzynski—or Gerson or Gonzales or any other pioneering practitioner whom vested interests would seek to destroy. It concerns the right of every innovative doctor to practice his profession without government interference, as long as he does no harm.

"The physician has but a single task," wrote Hippocrates, "to cure; and if he succeeds, it matters not a whit by what means he has succeeded."

Let the results speak for themselves!

We have strayed so far from the ideals on which our country was created that when the Founding Fathers look down on us now, they must be weeping with sorrow. We are governed by fools, ruled by corporations and multimillion-dollar foundations, lied to by the left as well as the right, and hoodwinked by hypocrisy at every turn. Once the proud Land of the Free and Home of the Brave, America has become the Land of the Lobbyist and Home of the Moral Coward.

Years ago Benjamin Rush, a physician and signer of the Declaration of Independence, warned, with far-reaching wisdom:

> Unless we put medical freedom into the Constitution, the
> time will come when medicine will organize an undercover
> dictatorship. To restrict the art of healing to one class of
> men, and deny equal privileges to others, will constitute the
> Bastille of medical science. All such laws are un-American
> and despotic.... The Constitution of this Republic should
> make special provisions for medical freedom as well as
> Religious Freedom.

EPILOGUE

In March 2011, a huge earthquake and tsunami crippled a nuclear power station in Fukushima, Japan, causing the worst nuclear disaster in history. Tests of well water in the area showed that radioactivity in the drinking water was more than one hundred times higher than the level considered safe, and a once-thriving fishing industry was wiped out.

After a typhoon passed through Japan, 3 years later in October 2014, the amount of radioactive water near the plant rose to record levels. Thousands of gallons of contaminated water are seeping into the Pacific Ocean, their environmental impact reaching far beyond Japan's shores.

We are committing global suicide on a scale unimagined by Rachel Carson, when she wrote in *The Sea Around Us*:

> It is a curious situation that the sea, from which life first arose, should now be threatened by the activities of one form of that life. But the sea, though changed in a sinister way, will continue to exist; the threat is rather to life itself.

That threat is now an imminent reality.

How many cancers do we need? How many shattered immune systems can we afford before our rampant exploitation of the planet is finally curbed? The evidence is all around us—in deformed frogs, dying fish, disappearing butterflies and bees, and trees whose branches have been denuded by acid rain.

The most urgent question facing us today is not climate change or whether the starving poor of the world can be fed, but whether man's folly will destroy the earth through environmental rapacity, fanatic religious terrorism, or both.

In the words attributed to Chief Seattle, head of the Suquamish tribe, in his famous speech of 1854:

> Where is the thicket? Gone.
> Where is the eagle? Gone.
> The end of living
> And the beginning of survival.

FAYE HUESTON

APPENDIX

CONTRAINDICATIONS AND CAUTIONS FOR THE GERSON THERAPY

While the Gerson Therapy has proven successful in treating a wide range of degenerative diseases, including cancer, it has been less effective with some, and has still to be tested with others.

A list of these conditions may be found on the Gerson website at **gerson.org**. The reader is advised to consult this list of precautions before determining if the therapy is their best option at this time, or if it might be better adopted in support of a medical protocol.

BIBLIOGRAPHY

Bellini, James. *High-Tech Holocaust*. David and Charles, 1989.

Bishop, Beata. *A Time to Heal*. 3rd ed. London: First Stone, Penguin Arkana, 1996. Available from the Gerson Institute, 4631 Viewridge Ave., San Diego, CA 92123.

Campbell, Joseph. *The Masks of God*. New York: Penguin Books, 1976.

Carson, Rachel L. *The Sea Around Us*. Oxford: Oxford University Press, 1953. Reprinted by permission of Frances Collin, Trustee.

Carson, Rachel L. *Silent Spring*. Houghton Mifflin, 1962. Reprinted by permission of Frances Collin, Trustee.

Christian Science *Science and Health, with Key to the Scriptures*. Boston: Trustees under the Will of Mary Baker G. Eddy, 1875.

Davison, Jaquie. *Cancer Winner*. Pierce City, MO: Pacific Press, 1977.

Davis, Devra. *The Secret History of the War on Cancer*. New York: Basic Books, 2007.

Davis, Lee N. *The Corporate Alchemists*. Middlesex, Great Britain: Maurice Temple Smith Ltd., 1984.

Eliot, George. *Middlemarch*. Oxford: Oxford University Press, 2008. Extract of 41 words. By permission of Oxford University Press.

Emord, Jonathan W. *The Rise of Tyranny*. Washington, D.C.: Sentinel Press, 2008.

Erlichman, James. *Gluttons for Punishment*. England: Peters, Fraser and Dunlop Ltd., 1986.

Food and Drug Administration *"FDA vs. The People of the United States, Five years of assault on 'self care.' "*: *The Jonathan Wright Legal Defense Fund*. Tacoma, Washington, May 1992.

Gerson, Max. *A Cancer Therapy: Results of Fifty Cases*. 1st ed. Del Mar, CA: Totality Books, 1958.

Hamilton, Edith. *The Greek Way.* New York: W. W. Norton, 1964.

Harburg, E.Y. Poem *"Diagnoses,"* *Rhymes for the Irreverent.* Glocca Morra Music, Administered by Next Decade Entertainment Inc., 1965. Used by permission of Harburg Foundation.

Hubbard, L. Ron. *Dianetics.* New York: Heritage House, 1950.

JAMA. *Journal of the American Medical Association.* Volume 132, number 11, Nov. 16, 1946.

JAMA. *Journal of the American Medical Association.* Volume 139, number 2, pp. 93-96, 1949.

Korzybski, Alfred. *Science and Sanity.* Germany: Institute of General Semantics, 1933.

LeShan, Lawrence. *You Can Fight for your Life.* New York: M. Evans & Co Inc., 1984.

Perry, Ted. Film script for Home (prod. by the Southern Baptist Radio and Television Commission, 1972), reprinted in Rudolf Kaiser, "Chief Seattle's Speech(es): American Origins and European Reception," in Recovering the Word: Essays on Native American Literature, ed. Brian Swann and Arnold Krupat (Berkeley: University of California Press, 1987), 525-530.

Piccardi, Giorgio. *The Chemical Basis of Medical Climatology.* Springfield, IL: Charles C. Thomas Publisher, Ltd., 1962.

Pollan, Michael. *In Defense of Food.* New York: The Penguin Press, 2008.

Randolph, Theron G. Randolph, MD. *Allergy: Your Hidden Enemy.* New York: Lippincott and Crowell, 1980.

Roa Bastos, Augusto. *I, The Supreme.* English translation. New York: Alfred A. Knopf, 1986.

St. Exupery, Antoine de. *Wind, Sand and Stars (Terre des Hommes).* Orlando: Harcourt Brace & Co., 1992.

Toynbee, Philip. *End of a Journey.* London: Bloomsbury Publishing Ltd., 1988.

Tributsch, Helmut. *When the Snakes Awake.* Cambridge: MIT Press, 1984.

Watson, Lyall. *Neophilia.* London: Hodder and Stoughton Ltd., 1989. Reproduced by permission of Pollinger Limited and the Estate of Lyall Watson.

Watson, Lyall. *Supernature.* London: Hodder and Stoughton Ltd., 1973. Reproduced by permission of Pollinger Limited and the Estate of Lyall Watson.

White, E. B. *Essays of E.B. White. Bedfellows.* Pg 86. New York: Harper Collins Books, 1976.

Wickes, Frances. *The Inner World of Choice.* Upper Saddle River, NJ: Prentice-Hall Inc., 1976.